I AM HERE

stories from a cancer ward

johannes klabbers

SCRIBE

Melbourne • London

Scribe Publications
18–20 Edward St, Brunswick, Victoria 3056, Australia
2 John St, Clerkenwell, London, WC1N 2ES, United Kingdom

First published by Scribe 2016

Typeset in 11.5/16.25 pt Adobe Caslon Pro by the publishers
Printed and bound in the UK by CPI Group (UK) Ltd, Croydon CR0 4YY

Scribe Publications is committed to the sustainable use of natural resources and the use of paper products made responsibly from those resources.

9781925321470 (AU paperback)
9781925228625 (UK paperback)
9781925307566 (e-book)

CiP records for this title are available from the National Library of Australia and the British Library

scribepublications.com.au
scribepublications.co.uk

Contents

Author's note

When I resigned from the university where I was a tenured academic, I had no idea what I was going to do next. Six months later, I began working full time as an unpaid pastoral-care intern at a major cancer hospital. In essence, the work was being there, talking to the patients, and listening to them if they wanted to talk. I had a Doctorate of Philosophy, a post-graduate teaching qualification, and a Bachelor's degree, but I was completely unprepared for the education I was about to receive, and I never worked harder than I did for the three qualifications I gained that year — a Basic, an Advanced, and a Post-advanced certificate in Pastoral Care. Each took three months to complete, with two-week breaks in between.

Once I'd passed the Basic unit, I was offered some paid pastoral work in the hospital during the breaks — and after I'd finished my internship, I frequently worked there as a casual pastoral worker when the hospital was short of staff, and during weekends and public holidays. (During most of those three years, I also worked a second job in computer support after hours to pay the rent.)

This book deals mainly with my experiences during that first year as a pastoral-care intern, although, in the writing, I have occasionally drawn on my experiences whilst working in the hospital in those subsequent years. The original idea for the book was to honour the people I encountered in the hospital—those who died and those who lived, at least for a while, and those who remain alive. What I would have liked to be able to say was *This is not my story, but theirs.* But as I was writing this book, I realised that no one can tell someone else's story. You can only tell your own story, and how it connects with other people's stories.

So this is a memoir: it is a book about how I experienced and remember the events; it does not attempt to provide a factual account. This is the story of how I was touched, challenged, and profoundly moved by my encounters with these people and the many others who did not make it into the book. In telling my own story and how I was changed by that year, I hope to have honoured their memories and perhaps given something back.

I have not named the hospital, and this book has not been endorsed by it. The book does not attempt to reflect the policies of the hospital, or the opinions of its employees. The names and personal details of the patients who I worked with, and their friends and families, have been changed in a genuine attempt to protect their identities, but all the people in the book are real.

The members of staff who appear in this book—the nurses and ward clerks, allied health staff, as well as my colleagues in pastoral care—are amalgamations or collages, with made-up names. Crucial though these people are in the care of the patients, and much as I respect and admire them, I felt I could be a little bit creative with those characters. All the same, I hope I have shown them appropriate respect.

Although I was enrolled in a Clinical Pastoral Education program, I have chosen to omit most of the mechanics of CPE, of which there is a rich tradition in Australia, the UK, and the US, and which I wished, for a time, to actively contribute to changing by making it more accessible to those with no religious beliefs. I hope this book can do something to help make that possible by demonstrating the richness and importance of a secular pastoral-care practice.

For a long time, I've held the view that it's sensible for people suffering unbearably from an incurable illness to legally request assistance to end their lives, as they can in my motherland and increasingly in other countries. I saw nothing in my three years of working in the hospital to make me think otherwise. I only aired my views on this subject on a couple of occasions in private conversation with one or two colleagues, and not at all with patients. Nor did I reveal that I was doing volunteer work for a right-to-die organisation—except to my head of department after finishing my internship. More recently, I worked part time for that organisation and actively advocated for end-of-life choices. I am continuing to think about this issue and how we can make it easier to talk to each other about death and dying. This will be the subject of my second book.

An Agnostic on Trial

Beginnings

I awake to grey skies on my first day as a pastoral-care intern, but my head is clear, and now that I am no longer working at the university I am surprised to find my mood is ... optimistic. It is difficult to imagine what this day and this week, let alone this year, will hold. But I am not afraid. *When you ain't got nothing, you ain't got nothing to lose*, as the song goes.

Pastoral care was not what I had in mind when I resigned my tenure at the university. Not that I had anything in mind, except to return to the real world, and to reinvent myself. I had no idea how I would do that or what I would do. What I did know was that I didn't want to spend my life trying to convince students that in order to make good art it has to be a matter of life and death. I knew that I wanted to spend my time with real human beings — as many different human beings as possible — and to find out if I could make a real difference in some of those people's lives. I knew that, at least in theory, students are real human beings, too, but after fifteen years, most of them seemed to me to be processing the material I fed them as mindlessly as the cows in the paddock near the university's experimental farm. But the cows were more interesting because part of the skin around the abdomen had been replaced with Perspex, so you could observe their digestive systems working.

I have walked to the hospital several times to see how long it will take and to make sure I'm not late and that I don't get lost. It takes a little less than an hour. The route takes me past the Melbourne Cricket Ground and through the lush Fitzroy Gardens where Captain Cook's cottage stands. Bought for 800 pounds by an Australian in 1933, it was transported brick by brick from Yorkshire and rebuilt here. Of more interest to me are an Aboriginal scarred tree and a statue of Diana the Huntress and her dogs. She wears a determined look, and not much else. Ah, the Victorians! In her right hand is a bow, whilst the other is pointing into the distance, as if to say 'Onward!'

Voluntarily relinquishing tenure, which is the holy grail for would-be academics the world over, is inconceivable for most people. But there is tenure, and then there is tenure in a small country town in rural Australia five-and-a-half hours drive from Sydney and four-and-a-half from Melbourne. There, tenure is like a soft prison sentence. Every second Thursday, they put two-and-a-half thousand dollars into your bank account, and the idea of that not happening anymore becomes terrifying. It is like an umbilical cord with which you are connected to an evil mother who sucks as much as she can out of you through the same channel that delivers the sweet milk.

The first day at the hospital begins under fluorescent lights in a windowless room with a sickly indoor plant in the corner. Our supervisor is a tall, good-looking man with lots of hair. He points out that we are all men, which is a first for the

Pastoral Care internship program. He tells us that he lost his father when he was four. I want to tell him that I, too, lost my father—when I was five—but the moment is gone. He is already dispensing information about cancer and the workings of the hospital. After a couple of hours it's time for a break. There is a celebratory morning tea, with cake and fruit and cheese. I eat too much cheese, a thing I always do when I'm anxious.

When I moved to the big smoke, I signed up as a volunteer in a large trauma hospital, visiting patients with a newspaper trolley. This was surprisingly demanding physical work for someone used to sitting behind a desk and driving his car to a lecture theatre. It was confronting emotionally as well, at times, but it was rewarding. I felt like I was making a difference to real people who were having a *really* hard time, even if all I could do for them was smile, make a joke, or have a chat about the weather or the football, and sell them a newspaper or a bar of chocolate. I always made sure I had plenty of good-quality chocolate on the trolley.

That was not nothing, and I loved doing it, but it was rare that I was able to do more. Boundaries were strongly emphasised in the volunteer training. We were not authorised to talk about 'big stuff' with patients. Deep and meaningful was out of bounds for pushers of newspaper trolleys. But whose job was it to talk to the patients about 'big stuff'? It didn't seem to be the medical staff's. It was clear that their job was to fix the physical problems and their aim was to get the patient well enough to be discharged. The psychologists? They were only called in when there was a possible mental-health problem. Although I did see the occasional rabbi or priest wandering around, they were looking for members of their 'flock'. They had neither the time nor the inclination to talk to people who did not belong to their particular religion, and vice versa probably. *So who talks to the non-believers*, I wondered?

On the form we filled in at the volunteer training day, there was a list of the areas in which volunteers were used. Next to 'Pastoral Care', it said: 'Note: only those who have completed the pastoral care training can volunteer for pastoral care.' One of the people who came and spoke to us that day was a reverend something or other who gave a brief talk about pastoral care. The penny dropped. In this secular hospital it was the believers who talked to the patients about meaning.

And now I am training in pastoral care. I furtively look around the room at the others. There are three other interns. One is younger than me, and he reminds me of my brother Patrick. The other two are older: one is talkative; the other, as quiet as a mouse. I am assuming everyone in the room is Christian. I plan to keep the information that I'm a non-believer under my hat for now, for fear of alienating people at the very beginning.

My initial enquiries about training in pastoral care did not meet with an encouraging response, probably because I made it clear I was a non-believer. 'Certainly, there would be no objection to you applying,' the acting head of the department at another hospital said in her curt email, 'but you would need a recommendation from your local priest.' She also explained that, for her, the training 'was most valuable in opening up ways of relating and sharing our faith in our creator God with not only patients.' Visions of hospital wards filled with ailing atheists being snubbed by holier-than-thou evangelists, so delirious with religious fervour that their grasp of basic grammar eluded them, haunted my dreams. A few days later, whilst attending a funeral, I eyed off the priest and imagined saying to him: 'I have a problem. I wonder if you would be prepared to give me a letter of recommendation to undergo pastoral-care training?'

'You're an atheist, and you want to train as a pastoral worker?' someone I was talking to at a party said and laughed. 'That's hilarious!'

'You should go and train in a cancer hospital,' someone who overheard the conversation, and who had been a patient, said to me. 'You'll have your work cut out for you there!'

At the end of the day, there is a tour of the facilities. Our guide is the sprightly senior pastoral worker—one of those who had interviewed me. She was the one least inclined to laugh at my jokes at the interview, but she is warm, forthcoming, and generous.

The interview was in a small but airy and light-filled room full of books—lots of books about Jesus and pastoral care, but Jung's *Man and his Symbols* was also there, and a complete set of Robert A. Johnson.

'First things first,' said the tall, good-looking man, who introduced himself as the head of department. 'Although a small stipend was advertised, this is no longer available. Are you still interested?' Lying awake during the night, I had wondered if they would be any more likely to give an internship to an atheist who was willing to forego the stipend.

'Well,' I said, 'it's funny you should say that. Because last night I thought: *What would happen if I walked in to the interview and said I'd be prepared to forego the stipend…?'* Laughter filled the room, and the ice was broken. For the next hour and a half I was grilled about everything from my faith and/or spirituality, to my work history and my reasons for wanting to be a pastoral worker, by three women and a man. I didn't have a lot of experience with religious people, but it seemed to me that, for Christians, they were surprisingly relaxed and generous, and all but one of them laughed heartily at my attempts at humour.

On the application form for the full-time one-year clinical pastoral-care internship offered at the hospital, in the section for the endorsement from my local priest, I wrote, after much agonising, in big letters: NOT APPLICABLE. In the biographical statement I carefully referred to myself as an agnostic, rather than as an atheist. But I felt I was going through the motions of applying more just to get it out of my system than anything else. It was an exorcism—that was it. If I never heard from them again, I would not have been surprised. But, several weeks later, I got a call asking me to come in for an interview.

In the interview, I stressed that I respected people of all religions, provided that they respected my right not to be religious, and that I was interested in how non-religious people make their lives meaningful. I might have mentioned Viktor Frankl, the Holocaust survivor and psychotherapist, who invented an alternative approach to psychoanalysis based on the search for meaning. I might have said I believed that the undeniable beauty and order of the universe is meaningful. I might even have said that I found consolation in the idea that there are eleven dimensions and ten-to-the-power-of-five-hundred universes, as predicted by some quantum physicists.

That same afternoon, when I received the phone call offering me an internship, I was stunned. It was surreal. For the next twelve months, when people asked: 'What do you do?' I would say: 'I'm a pastoral worker in a cancer hospital.'

The hospital consists of two separate buildings, one dating from just after the war and the other from the early seventies, joined in a haphazard way by a myriad of stairs, ramps, and corridors. We are introduced to some of the staff on each of the wards, of which there are five. One is the day unit, one is for young people, and another is the general surgery ward. The other two wards are more or less dedicated to specific cancers — one for the head, neck and lungs; the other, for the blood cancers: leukaemia, lymphoma, and myeloma.

The prevailing philosophy seems to be that there is only one way to learn pastoral care, and that is by doing it. Back in the office, our supervisor wants to know which ward we would prefer to work on. 'Because,' he says with more than a hint of glee, 'tomorrow we throw you in at the deep end!'

I have no idea.

The next day, we re-enter the windowless room to find out which wards we have been assigned to. I've been given the head, neck, and lung-cancer ward. The four of us leave the office together. The hospital is a short walk down the road. Waiting at the lifts, we are anxious. None of us has ever done anything remotely like this before. But this is what we've come here to do, and it seems now is when we're going to be doing it.

These are the slowest lifts in the known universe. 'Good luck!' we say nervously to each other, as it stops at each ward.

Mine is the penultimate floor. The quietest of my colleagues, says 'Good luck!' and touches me on the shoulder. As the lift doors close behind me, I realise there will be no one left to wish him good luck when he gets to the top floor. 'Good luck!' I say to the closed lift doors. A passing orderly looks at me strangely.

I swallow hard as I enter for the first time what is to be 'my' ward. Apparently I'm now a pastoral worker. I'm wearing a badge that says so. On it is a picture of me trying to smile at the sullen security guard, whose job it is to take the pictures for the IDs. I guess this is the deep end that my supervisor was talking about. I disinfect my hands and enter the ward via the squeaky swinging doors. At the front desk is Carla, the nurse in charge: a tall, fit-looking woman in her late twenties, with undyed sensible hair and shoes, she exudes competence. Carla remembers me from yesterday, and suggests a couple of patients I might like to go and 'have a chat' with.

The layout of the wards was breezily explained yesterday, but finding bed C in room 5 takes longer than it should. And now I must be looking at what I am thinking of at this point as 'my patient': a man around my own age with half his face missing and a tube going into a hole where his nose once was. He is vomiting into a bag. The two young women on either side of the bed could be his daughters. One of them is sobbing loudly, and, judging from her face, she's been doing this for a long time. A small girl is playing happily on the floor near the bed with a large green dinosaur, apparently oblivious to what's going on. The other woman speaks in what sounds like Russian to the man, who is clearly in no state to 'have a chat' with me. I am confused.

Why did Carla send me to see this patient?

The sobbing woman keeps looking at me and saying: 'It's terrible. It's awful.' I feel awkward and completely useless. I sit down on the chair and I pat her arm. It's all I can think of. I stay there for a while. I look at the little girl playing, and I say to the sobbing woman: 'She's beautiful, isn't she?'

'Yes. She's beautiful, but …' and then she says something I can't understand because of her heavy accent and the sobbing.

I say my goodbyes with a heavy heart.

'All the best. I'll come and see how you're going tomorrow …'

I wave at the little girl, and she gives me a weak smile.

I find the day room. This is where patients and their families can make a cup of tea or coffee and watch TV if they want to get out of their room for a while. Luckily, it is empty. I stand there and look at the city of Melbourne. There is the MCG. There is the Rod Laver Tennis Arena. I make a note on my ward list about the Russian patient. The second name on the list with an asterix next to it is 'Eugene'.

Eugene

'Hello … Eugene, is it?' Sitting in the bed is a balding middle-aged man, with a significant gut on him. He looks up from his mobile phone for a moment and nods.

'I'm Johannes from Pastoral Care.'

'Yes?' he says almost inaudibly.

'I'm just here to introduce myself and … to have a chat with you … if you like.'

Eugene looks pale, tired, unwell, and unhappy. 'OK. What kind of chat d'you wanna have?' he asks wearily, without really looking at me.

'Well … we can talk about the cricket. Or … the football, or we can have a deep and meaningful conversation … Whatever you like …!' I say cheerfully.

Eugene immediately launches into a monologue about the lack of quality in the recent performances of the Australian cricket team in the one-day series. I don't really know much about cricket, but I read the headlines, so I can more or less hold up my end of a conversation about it.

'It didn't take them long to drop Ricky Ponting!' I offer.

'Well, Ponting was never much of a player in the short form of the game,' Eugene ponders.

I wouldn't have a clue, but I've read *How to Win Friends and Influence People.*

'So you think Ponting is more suited to test cricket?' This is followed by an extended analysis of the relative merits or otherwise of the Australian captain and vice-captain, with very little input required from me. I am sitting by the side of the bed, so Eugene is facing away from me, and he seems to be looking out of the window. It is as if he is talking to no one in particular. His room has a great view of St. Patrick's cathedral, so perhaps he is addressing a higher power, as sports fans often seem to do.

I take the opportunity presented by a few moments of silence and say: 'So, that was the cricket. What about football?'

As if on cue, Eugene embarks on a rant about the apparent controversy over whether the captain of St. Kilda, Nick

Riewoldt, is gay or not. I'm not aware of any such controversy, and say so.

'It's been all over the papers!' Eugene exclaims incredulously. He gives me a sideways glance. I have to think quickly. As an ex-pusher of a newspaper trolley in a place where people have a lot of time on their hands, I was subjected to more than one homophobic diatribe in response to whatever was in the *Herald Sun* at the time.

'Maybe that's why Riewoldt didn't have a good season last year,' I say quickly, 'because everyone speculating about his sexuality was worrying him?'

'Hmmm … I don't know.'

Eugene turns to make eye contact for the first time, and says with a wink that he is 'buy-sexual'. I don't get that this is a joke at first. I hear 'bisexual' and don't notice the wink, so I ask if it's an issue for him.

'I'm single, so if I want sex I have to go and buy it …' he says, and laughs. I am still confused. 'So … I'm a buy-sexual!' he says triumphantly.

I laugh heartily at this, not because I think it's at all funny, but because the tension of my first day on the ward is broken, and he had me fooled. Eugene is pleased that he made me laugh. 'Didn't they tell you I was a joker?'

'No, they didn't. But they should've!' The mood has lightened considerably. I feel buoyant. I've managed to cheer up a patient! Does this mean I'm doing pastoral care now? Or did *he* cheer *me* up? I never got this far with anyone when I was pushing the newspaper trolley, although an old man told me about his Holocaust experiences once when I said he was lucky because he got the last copy of the *Jewish News*.

'So, that leaves money and religion,' Eugene says breezily.

'I don't like talking about money so ...'

'... Religion.'

'Well, I'm an agnostic,' I offer.

'Oh, I see. What does that mean?'

'It means you're not entirely sure.'

On the application form, I'd described myself as an agnostic rather than a non-believer, and this is the basis on which I was offered the position, so I feel I'd better stick to it. In any case, to be perfectly honest, I'm not entirely sure about anything.

'Well, that's me as well, then. I thought it means that you don't believe.'

'That's an atheist.'

'Oh.' He looks at me seriously now. 'Well, if there is a God, I wish he would tell me why this happened to me ... Why me?'

'You wish that God would tell you why ... you got the disease?'

'Yeah. Or, if it was just that my number was up, that he would just tell me that,' Eugene sighs.

'Maybe between now and the next time I come to visit, you could think about how you would talk to God, if there is one, about what is happening to you?'

'Thank you. I will do that.'

'Thanks, Eugene. I will try to come and see you tomorrow.'

'That would be good.' He looks weary again.

The next day, I get talking to James in the bed opposite Eugene. He is a GP in his mid-seventies with advanced bladder cancer. We talk about politics. When I say it is time for me to go, he asks: 'So, what's your faith?'

'I'm an agnostic.'

'I'm an atheist!'

'OK, and so you're a rationalist!' I say smiling.

He looks askance and smiles in a non-committal way. I try to talk to him about quantum entanglement, but I am a bit tired and vague today.

The sign of the father

Eugene tells me he's a mechanic. He used to work with his dad. He was a mechanic, too. They had their own garage.

'We made a lot of money,' he says casually.

I am keen to try and avoid a conversation about money. My Dutch forefathers loved to talk about money, but I'm an Australian now.

'Do you have a good relationship with your father?'

Eugene says that he used to feel like his dad was watching over him, but lately he hasn't felt like that.

'So, he is no longer alive?'

'No. He died.'

'A long time ago, or recently?'

'About ten years ago,' Eugene says sadly.

'I see. And was it sudden?'

'Yes.'

'And how did it make you feel, your dad passing away suddenly like that?'

'Not very good.'

His face doesn't reveal any sign of him crying, but I watch a tear fall out of his eye.

My own father passed away suddenly at the age of 45. I was 19. We lived in different countries and didn't see each other very often, but the death of the father is a momentous event in a man's life. I immediately feel a connection with Eugene.

'I lost my dad when I was 19,' I say. We are both silent for quite a while. 'What was the worst thing for you about losing your dad?' I ask.

He thinks for a moment. 'Not having a chance to say what I would have liked to have said to him …'

What I would have liked to say to Eugene was that the fact that someone is dead doesn't mean you can't say the things you would like to say to them. What I would like to say is: *Would you like to say it to him now?* But I don't feel confident enough. I think: *Maybe this is enough pastoral work for one visit …*

The uncertainty principle

The next day, the bed opposite Eugene is empty. Eugene says, 'They moved James into a single room.'

'Why?'

'Don't know.' He pulls a face. 'Maybe he got sick of my whingin'!'

'Poor you!' I say. 'You'll miss him.'

'It's OK,' he says. 'It's good for me! I can go for a walk and visit him.'

I go and see James every day. We have numerous conversations about everything from art to the merits of the Bulldogs and quantum physics. 'But James,' I say to him one day, 'somewhere the Bulldogs are winning! There are eleven dimensions and ten-to-the-power-of-five-hundred universes all running in parallel.'

'Really?' he says drily. 'That seems like a lot. Are you sure?'

I'm not sure, and I don't answer, but every night we spend hours and hours in an irrational universe where everything is fluid and random, and where Heisenberg's uncertainty principle reigns. 'What we observe is not nature itself,' Heisenberg wrote, 'but nature exposed to our method of questioning.' Perhaps it is when we are asleep and the observer is unconscious that we exist in the other possible dimensions and universes that some quantum theorists say are happening.

James and I grow fond of each other—no longer carefully polite, but genuinely warm. He is always pleased to see me. 'Come in … come in …' he says when he opens his eyes and sees me standing at the door trying to work out if he is asleep.

After Eugene is moved to a different floor and he can no longer visit, James asks about him. I can't think of two men with less in common, but he always says: 'Have you seen Eugene today? Is he still in? How is he?'

And Eugene enquires after James, and I pass on regards from one to the other.

Punishment

Some days are equal parts strangeness and uncertainty. Today is an odd day. There is no flow. None of the patients wants to talk to me. I feel kind of deflated. Going to see James was no help. He's usually good for an hour of conversation, but he was off the ward having a procedure done, and then he was fast asleep when I went in to see him this afternoon.

Eugene had told the worker on his new ward that he would like me to come and see him. He broke down within minutes of me getting there. But when I asked what was bothering him, he told me to 'piss off' so he could do his lunch order.

I feel useless. At lunch I seek out the most senior pastoral worker on my team and complain about Eugene's rudeness. She reminds me that people being treated in the hospital are often affected by the drugs they are taking, and sometimes the drugs they are on are changed and they may experience mood swings.

And then there is Michael.

Michael, recently admitted with rapidly advancing lung cancer, was the subject of a medical emergency on my ward this morning. I go to check on him in the afternoon. He has that grey look of someone who is not getting enough oxygen.

'Hello, I'm Johannes from Pastoral Care. I'm here to see how you are feeling after your emergency this morning.'

'Oh, I was sick this morning, was I?' He looks so immensely sad behind his oxygen mask.

'Yes.'

On this ward, some of the male patients can be a bit rough and ready, and sometimes angry or aggressive, or both. On an intellectual level, I can appreciate that they are angry about their disease, but on a human level I feel sad, and I don't seem to be able to help being a little bit offended when they don't want to talk to me.

Michael is rough and ready, but he is not angry. He is sad and afraid. He says, 'There is not much hope.'

'Why do you feel like there is no hope, Michael?'

This is a stupid question, and I know it almost as soon as I've said it. I feel like an idiot. He looks at me with big eyes. I think he says something about being punished. Because of the oxygen mask his voice is muffled, and I don't quite hear him properly.

'Did you say you feel like you are being punished?'

But the moment is gone, and Michael says he doesn't really want to talk about it.

'Can I come back and see you again?'

'OK. If you want.'

I am sweating. Michael will never know it, but later I realise that he taught me an invaluable lesson. *Pay attention! Be there. Never go into automatic pilot. Sometimes you have to do a lot of work for a very small return.*

This felt like a little victory. I asked a stupid question. He didn't punish me. I have won the tiniest of battles in getting him to agree to another visit. But all I feel is sad. Sad and useless. Maybe if Michael was able to talk to me about it, he would feel better—or maybe not. I have to trust him. I can only help him if he wants to be helped. And he has agreed that I can come back, so next time I can look for an opportunity to ask him about punishment.

The impressionist

When I come back to the hospital after a weekend off, Michael is gone. Maybe he has been moved to a different ward. I check all the ward lists, but his name is not there. He may have been discharged to a hospice or a local hospital. Or he could have died. He was close. Sometimes someone's name and 'RIP' appears on the whiteboard in the ward's changeover room, but Michael's is not there. I might be able to find out what happened to him by consulting the patients' records system, as some of my colleagues do, but I don't. What difference would it make to him? The difference it makes to me is that I am more aware than ever that this conversation with a person may be the only opportunity I will ever have to connect with them. I need to be more present to that reality.

In my journal, I usually don't bother with capitals. I write:

> james was very jovial today. he even has some colour in his face now. his skin was almost translucent before. he complained humorously when i said i only had a few minutes because i had to go to a meeting. he told me again he is an atheist, was he worried i had forgotten? i said, i might turn you into an agnostic! i gave him an article by david bohm about quantum physics.

James sighs. 'You know, sometimes I curse myself.'
'Oh?'
'I don't know why I didn't have it checked out earlier. I am a doctor. I should have!' He frowns. 'And it would have been

easy for me. But I just didn't. I don't know why. And then it was too late!'

I tell him I'm a doctor, too — in fine arts — and that it didn't help my art making. James loves art, and he thinks it's marvellous that I have a doctorate in fine art. But he grows despondent when he is trying to tell me about one of his favourite painters, the impressionist … and can't think of the name. I name all the impressionists and post-impressionists I can think of …

'Manet? Monet?'

But I am mostly interested in contemporary art, and, as a practitioner of anything except painting, I've never taken much interest in it. Also, impressionism is probably the dullest of all the movements, but James looks pained. I keep trying.

'… Gaugin? Van Gogh? Degas? … er … Descartes? Hang on, no, he was a philosopher.'

James looks at me quizzically.

'Sorry, James, one old painting is much like another to me.'

He says sadly, 'I think I might have a sleep now, Johannes, if you don't mind.'

'Of course. See you, James.'

You can build up a wonderful ongoing relationship with a person being treated in the hospital, and then you come back after a day off to find them gone. They have been suddenly discharged without notice, or they have died, and you didn't get a chance to say goodbye. You didn't expect them to be gone and you weren't prepared. You miss them, and you wonder how they are.

James has been on the waiting list for a bed at one or other of the hospices, and I have the good fortune of being in the foyer when he is being wheeled out one morning, on his way to the ambulance to be taken to the hospice, so I am able to say a hurried farewell. In my bag is a book about impressionist painters I've borrowed from the library. I would have liked to look through it with him. Maybe we could have found out the name of that elusive impressionist.

Scratch my back for a penny

Ben looks terrible. He's distressed and agitated. He ripped out his tubes during the night, and it was a job for the nurses reinserting them. He was drifting in and out of consciousness, but he fought with them tooth and nail.

Ben was admitted yesterday after having been in remission from lung cancer for a number of years. I am expecting a very sick man, because this is what the nurse in charge said in the ward meeting. But 'very sick' can mean a lot of different things. It can mean 'too unwell for pastoral care', and I must admit I've looked in on very sick people, decided there was nothing I could do for them, and left again. But there is always something you can do. You can sit with them. You can always sit with them. No one is going to say, 'What are you doing there?' You're the pastoral worker. You are doing your work, even if you are 'just' sitting with someone. And if they are very sick, chances are they're not going to tell you they don't want you there. But I've not had much luck connecting with people who are as sick as Ben sounds. And the sound, as I walk towards his room, is not like coughing—it is like someone is trying to expel the whole of their lungs.

Sharon, his daughter, is with him. She is my age. People's ages are important in the hospital. If they are younger than you, you think: *They are too young! This shouldn't be happening to them at that age.* If they are older than you, you feel sorry that they have to go through this at their age. If they are about the same age as you, you think: *There is absolutely no rhyme or reason as to why this isn't me. This disease is just completely random.*

I introduce myself and ask Ben how he's going. He is barely conscious, but somehow he manages to acknowledge my presence and form the words 'not happy' with his mouth. There is not enough air available for his voice box to make any actual sound.

Sharon is stroking his hand, saying, 'It's OK. It's all right, Dad.'

She looks weary. Her clothes are crumpled. There is a mattress in the corner of the room. She's been there all night.

I say, 'How are you coping?'

'OK ... I guess.'

I am so completely out of my depth that I wish a hole would open up in the ground and swallow me. *What do I have to offer these people?* I mutter something about the importance of support and strength. I do not say 'hope.' Sharon nods patiently.

'We knew it was coming,' she says. 'He knew it, we knew it. But you're still not prepared.' She smiles a half smile, almost apologetic.

Ben proceeds to have another bad coughing fit. That is, his body wants to cough, but Ben doesn't have the strength.

He seems to be drowning in phlegm and slime. There is fear in his eyes. He gives his daughter a pleading look. She runs out of the room to get a nurse. I put my hand in Ben's hand, where Sharon's hand was.

Sharon comes back with a nurse called Rick. Like most of the nurses in this hospital, he is in the prime of his life, straight backed, calm, and practical. He speaks to Ben as if to a child, or a kitten that's been sharpening its nails on the couch. 'Ben, this is why you have to leave the tubes in, you see, so they can drain the fluid,' he says gently.

I wonder what Rick does after work. I dated a nurse once, and sometimes she would fall in a heap when she came home, and sometimes she would want to party. But I have no idea what it's like to be a nurse, except it seems as if a significant number of the problems a nurse deals with involve unruly liquids: fluids that need to go into the body somehow, or bodily fluids escaping from the body, or finding their way to parts of the body where they shouldn't be.

Suddenly the room is full as two large people, Ben's sister, Margaret, and her husband, John, enter. Margaret is wearing a cheerful dress with large purple flowers, and John an ill-fitting brown suit and an incongruous tie. She stares incredulously at Ben and weeps quietly. Sharon explains that Margaret hasn't seen Ben since he was admitted. She suggests going into the day room to cry and have a coffee.

I don't know whether to go with them to the day room or stay with Ben. Rick's calm presence has settled him, and the coughing fit has ended. Margaret starts telling me about their sister who died on New Year's Eve, so I follow everyone out.

'Ben was at the funeral,' Margaret says. 'He didn't look

well then, but I'm shocked to see the state he's in now!'

She sits down and weeps soundlessly. I put a box of tissues near her. She dries her eyes and blows her nose elaborately, as country people are wont to do. She shakes her head when Sharon offers to make her coffee. Everyone sits except me. There are not enough chairs. I stand awkwardly.

Suddenly, Margaret says through her tears, 'He used to say "Margaret … scratch my back for a penny?"'

Everyone looks at her.

'But he never paid me!'

We all laugh heartily, and the sadness and tension is momentarily dispelled.

'He was a loveable lout,' she says, using the past tense.

'What sort of things did he used to do?' I ask.

'Oh, he was terrible! You would get so angry with him, and you would say, *I'm never doing anything for him again*. But then, he had this way, and he would ask you, and you would end up doing it anyway.'

The conversation evolves into one about smoking. Ben was an unrepentant smoker all his life. He asked Sharon for a cigarette only yesterday.

'He used to smoke chop chop,' Margaret says, 'I would say "I wish you wouldn't smoke that. You don't know what's in it!" But he used to say, "Something has to kill you!"'

'Yes,' I agree, 'but there is death and death.'

Everyone nods. We all talk about how long it is since we each gave up smoking, and John, who has been silent up to now, unbuttons his jacket and leans forward.

'Players!' he says with a nostalgic look. 'Camels …' He thinks for a while. 'Lucky Strike!'

'Number Six,' I offer. 'In packets of ten … Did you have them here?'

I imagine this same scene being played out weeks or months later in a draughty church hall in a country town, over ham and chicken sandwiches and mini sausage rolls, washed down with Crown lager.

Everyone is calm now. We sit together in silence, each with our own thoughts. I think about my father, who was a heavy smoker all his life. I've been thinking a lot about him since I've been working here. But he didn't die the long drawn-out death of cancer. He died quickly and painlessly from a brain haemorrhage, although he was still very young — much younger than I am now. I used to think, *Poor old bastard.* And now I think, *Too young! Too young.* Just like all the old people said when he died.

'I have to go,' I say after a while. John shakes my hand enthusiastically, as if I've just bought some of his sheep. Everyone thanks me.

'What for? I didn't do anything,' I say to my supervisor at the end of the day.

He strokes his beard and looks thoughtful. 'You were *there* for them,' he says. 'You could have made your excuses when they went into the day room, but you didn't. You stayed with them.'

It seems I am being a pastoral worker.

The inventory

Since talking with Michael I've had a growing suspicion that Eugene thinks he's got cancer because he has sinned. He told me he's a lapsed Catholic, and he keeps hinting that maybe he is being punished for something.

In Alcoholics Anonymous, one of the twelve steps is a confessional procedure called 'The Inventory'. This is where you write down all the bad things you've done in your life. They call this 'making a searching and fearless moral inventory of ourselves in which we admit, to ourselves, and to another human being, the exact nature of our wrongs'.

But, even though I am a non-believer, and an ex-alcoholic, I do think having a conversation with God can be useful. It doesn't matter if you're not a believer. It doesn't matter whether anyone is actually listening. It can function as a way of working through or processing the past—and the present—and coming to terms with what is happening to you, in the same way as the AA inventory.

But I have no idea how to raise it with Eugene. I wish I could say, *I can hear your confession.* Why not? I am still technically a Catholic. I took my First Communion, although I was never confirmed and I couldn't name more than about three or four of the ten commandments, and none of the mortal sins. Maybe I should ask if he would like a priest to come.

When I tell Eugene that I have to go, he says, pointing at the church outside, 'I have to work out how to forgive him …'

'You mean God?'

'Yes.'

'What do you want to tell him?'

There is silence for a few minutes. Tears well up in his eyes. He asks in a small voice, 'What did I do?'

Double Dutch

A tiny shape in a foetal position completely covered by a hospital blanket, Kelly is new on my ward. She's asleep when I check in on Room 8, but Ron, her husband, is sitting by the bed. His rough and ready appearance suggests a hard life. His skin is thick and weathered—brown, like leather. She's not feeling well at all, he tells me.

Ron seems annoyed, or maybe he's bored or tired—or all three. They're from Griffith in New South Wales. Kelly came by air ambulance, but Ron had to drive the whole 500 kilometres, at the end of which he must have had to bore his way through the Melbourne CBD and find a parking space. On top of the hospital blanket is a crocheted throw of cheerful primary colours. I've been surprised by how few patients bring anything of their own to the hospital.

I mention to Ron I lived in Wagga Wagga for fifteen years, and his face lights up a little. It's only a hundred or so kilometres from Griffith. He takes my card with a big hairy hand, and after glancing at it, asks if I'm Dutch.

'Yes, I am!' I say enthusiastically, and, having only recently bitten the bullet and taken out citizenship, 'Dutch/Australian. Came out when I was 22 …'

He says his son-in-law's name is Johannes, too.

'OK … is he …?'

'He's Dutch,' he says, with a tone of resignation.

There must be people in the world who are yet to encounter a Dutch person, but there can't be many of them. Everyone I meet has either had good experiences with Dutch people, or really, *really* bad ones. It means that when my being Dutch comes into the conversation, I often get a knowing look.

'Right. What's he like?'

'He's an idiot.'

He looks at me to see how I will react. I laugh. Laughing is the only response.

He almost smiles, and ventures, 'No offence …'

'None taken. There are plenty of them!'

Ron, being from Griffith, is the best part of a day's drive from home, in the big smoke, which he hates — or purports to hate. I know that feeling. I survived for many years in a small country town by denying that there was much in the city that I missed. But Ron is Griffith born and bred, as was his father, and his father before him.

We talk about fathers. He tells me about his life as a boy on the farm. His father treated him like a slave, he says. I ask him if he has ever spoken to his father about how he feels about being treated like that when he was a boy. He says nothing. He looks at me as if I am an idiot, too, and perhaps I am.

I notice an elderly lady in a chair by the window glancing across at us a few times as I am talking to Ron, and after I've said goodbye to him and promised to call back later, I go over and say hello.

My ward sheet says her name is Iris, and she is 86. She smiles at me sadly when I ask if I can sit with her.

She says, 'Yes, yes.'

Iris tells me she is going home soon. Yes. Her daughter is coming from Queensland to look after her for two months. Yes. I guess that's all she's got left. I'm unsure at first if I am hearing it right but, yes, Iris punctuates each sentence with the word 'yes'. She tells me she has cancer in her nose. Yes.

There are ten-to-the-power-of-five-hundred universes, and three hundred and sixty-seven different kinds of cancer. Some are said to be worse than others, but for me the worst kind is always the one that whoever it is I'm talking to at the time is telling me about. And I am only just beginning to realise that there is nothing of any use whatsoever that you can say in response.

There's no point saying to Iris, 'That's terrible.' It is clear from her sad face that she knows that. And you can't go around saying 'I'm sorry' to everyone you talk to all day every day, although when I am, when I feel it—and for whatever reason you don't always—I do say, 'I'm sorry.'

But what you can do—and what you must do—is not flinch, not avert your gaze, remain present. Be yourself, whatever that means. Being authentic is what they call it in clinical pastoral-speak. I don't know if they've read Heidegger, but what it means here is, don't bullshit. When you are training as a pastoral worker in a cancer hospital, the first thing you learn is that a person who has been diagnosed with a terminal illness has a supercharged bullshit detector. They have no time for it. So don't say you're sorry if you're not.

Iris says, 'You have beautiful blue eyes. Yes.'

'That's what Anna says!' I am beginning to feel more like myself.

Iris asks who Anna is. When I tell her, she says dreamily, 'I bet she's beautiful. Yes?'

'Yes, she is. Every morning when I wake up, I look at her and feel happy.'

We have a moment together, Iris and I. Yes.

Not dead yet

Geoffrey was the subject of a medical emergency today, but he's feeling better now, and his whole family has come to support him. The ward is overflowing with people of all ages and shapes and sizes. They are his children and grandchildren and their children and his siblings, and all of their partners and their children as well, it seems. They are talking in the corridors. They are sitting and standing in the day room watching TV and making cups of tea and coffee for each other, and laughing.

And Geoffrey is sitting up in bed, relishing all the attention. The mood is surprisingly upbeat for a cancer ward, and it affects the nurses and the orderlies and the cleaners. Everyone is smiling, and even the grumpiest nurse of them all, the one with the tic, looks like she is having to work at suppressing a smile. When she walks past, I suppress the urge to say, *Go on!*

Who are all these lovely people, and why are they happy? They are happy because Geoffrey is not dead yet—and they have hope. And here, I think, is a crucial difference between atheists: there are the passive nihilists, and the ones who believe in truth and beauty—even if it is unknowable and cannot be understood. There is a kind of atheist who has doubt, but who is also a radical optimist. There *is* meaning. There *is* a point, a *punctum*, somewhere in all the apparent truth and beauty and awe we experience in the ten-to-the-power-of-five-hundred universes and the eleven dimensions.

Meanwhile the passive nihilist is marooned in a cold and dark meaningless universe where life is just an accident, and so is beauty, and so is compassion. Where truth is something that must be demonstrated and repeatable. But, I for one, don't want to live in your cold, dark universe and get sucked into your black hole. So many things that are delightful and beautiful are irrational. And this is what Geoffrey, and the others I was yet to meet, taught me.

Each day, unencumbered by illness and mostly free of pain, I walk to work in the sunshine by the Yarra. Even on dull, cold mornings in the approaching winter, I am conscious of my extreme good fortune. I also know it is by the hair of my chinny-chin-chin and the skin of my yellow country teeth that I made it here. I'm more than just a lucky dog, although I certainly am one.

It was around that time that I started coming out as a non-believer and saying 'and I don't believe in isms either.' And sometimes I used to say to my colleagues and fellow interns, who are all Christians of various flavours, except one who is a Buddhist, 'I'm an atheist who believes in miracles.' This is because in the ten-to-the-power-of-five-hundred universes things that appear miraculous happen all the time, although in quantum physics the concept of time itself is highly problematic.

Day duty

All full-time pastoral-care department staff, including interns, take turns to do day duty. Everyone is assigned one of the days of the week. If you're on day duty, you come in at 8.00 am—when the on-call worker finishes. You print the ward lists, attend to any messages that have come in overnight, and carry the department pager (in addition to your own) that day. It is your job to respond to all Medical Emergency Team (MET) calls, wherever they happen in the hospital. The aim is to have a pastoral worker available at all MET calls during normal hours. A MET call can be upsetting for family members who might be visiting or staying with the ill person, because it is announced on the public-address system, and people come rushing from everywhere with equipment and serious expressions on their faces, and visitors have to leave the room.

My day-duty day is Monday, and it is Monday morning. No sooner have I walked into the office and taken off my coat than the public-address system springs into life and begins to crackle … *Attention. Respond Em EE Tee. Bed 2 Ward 5. Repeat. Respond Em EE Tee. Bed 2 Ward 5.* And I am back in the increasingly crisp autumn morning to walk from the office, which is located in a separate building next door, to the hospital.

Ward 5 is not my ward, and I haven't met Amala, but she's been mentioned at handover a couple of times. She is a Muslim woman with no English and a large family, several of whom are always in attendance.

I spend a bit of time with her husband, and her son and

daughter. They have been sleeping in their mother's room, taking it in turns to comfort her when necessary. They say they are OK. I offer my card, and say if they need someone to sit with her or with them, or someone to talk to, we are there for them. They thank me, but say very formally and politely, 'It is not needed.'

On an impulse, I put my hand on the shoulder of the sad-looking husband, and they both turn their heads and look at me with a sad smile. I just stay there for a while, and it seems meaningful and good—and it is. Who needs words?

An unnecessary stain

There was a moment of supreme happiness early today, walking in the autumn morning light in this great city, when I was thinking, *Why would you want to be anywhere else in the world? This is my home. And it is my home because I chose it.* I don't live here because my parents live here or conceived me here, or because this is where I happened to land, my boat stranded on some beach around here.

All those refugees who come here on rickety boats on treacherous seas, we should be rolling out the fucking red carpet for them. Every year there should be a New Australian of the Year award for the person who went through the most hardship to get here. Economic refugees, my arse. They want to work, but there are no jobs. But that's because companies can make bigger profits importing things from China.

Why would you want to do anything else with your life?

But that was before I visited Eugene. I wanted to tell him about the eleven dimensions, but he wants to tell me about his travels in South-East Asia, and there ensues a monologue about how much everything costs, where to get a decent feed at a reasonable price in Bangkok … and the bus from the airport to downtown is only … etc, etc. … and the girls! … something something … I can't remember. I must've blocked it out because, as he is telling me all this, it gradually dawns on me: *He was a sex tourist.* I feel stupid.

At lunch I go for a walk in the Fitzroy Gardens instead of having my sandwich in the lunchroom with the others, as I usually do. Lunch is an important part of the day where everyone gets a chance to forget about whatever they have had to deal with that morning and/or will encounter that afternoon. It is like a decompression chamber. Talking about work is banned. Laughing is encouraged, and no joke or pun is too stupid or tasteless.

But today I don't want to laugh. I need to see Diana the Huntress. I want to counter Eugene's absent but implicit confession, which was so disturbing and distasteful to me, with the life-size image of female pride and defiance that stands just outside the conservatory in the gardens.

'Even if I could go back, I'm useless down there now,' Eugene had said. Here is a man with a stoma, dying of cancer, who boasts about his millions and having sex with women living in poverty in a third world country, mourning the loss of his virility.

And then I remember what I thought about this morning, walking to the hospital. This, too, is part of the work. This is my work, and I chose it. And that was then and this is now. And here, now, my job is to support this man who is dying and whose millions are useless to him; in fact, they are a burden, as is his past. There is a human being in there. I think I can see him. *Just.*

A poor prognosis

The prognosis for Kelly is poor. She is going back home to Griffith for palliative care. Euphemisms for death abound in the hospital. 'Limited treatment options' or 'poor prognosis' means you're going to die at some point in the not-too-distant future.

Plenty of people die in the hospital, although almost everyone prefers it if the dying happens somewhere else. But some people die suddenly, unexpectedly—and others take a long time to die. Sometimes a person is not well enough to be moved and it is decided to let them die in the hospital.

Ron left for Griffith a few days ago. Kelly will go back with the air ambulance. Kelly and I have grown close. We have nothing in common except our age, a family connection with a Dutch person, and the fact that for fifteen years I lived and worked one hundred kilometres down a dusty road from where she's lived all her life.

We sit together for the last time. She has no more than a few months to live, at best, but she is happy.

'Glad to be off home?'

'Yeah, I reckon! Back to me chooks and the grandkids.'

'I'll miss your smiling face!'

'Thanks for everything you've done for me.'

'That's no worries! I wish I could have done more.'

'That's all right. You've been great. Really!'

She looks me directly in the eye to make sure I've understood.

I've actually done nothing except sit with her, and talk about the weather and ask her about life back in Griffith. But she enjoyed telling me about her grandchildren, and how much she loves them, John especially.

'Will John be there when you get home?'

'No … he'll be away at school. But he might come home for the weekend. I'm so looking forward to seeing him.'

Her voice has a strange, high pitch. It's been like that for the whole time I've known her, but even more so now, and it blends with the steady rushing sound of the oxygen that flows into her because her lungs are less and less able to do the work of extracting it from the air she breathes.

Prayer

Some pastoral workers talk the talk. They meticulously check the patient notes before going to see someone, and they know all about the different kinds of cancers you can have. Words like *squamous* and *choroidal* roll off their tongues. I know nothing about cancer, beyond the fact that there are three hundred and fifty-seven different kinds. I don't know what they are, and I don't want to know. 'Talk to *me*—not to my cancer,' a patient said to me.

A person is called a patient because there is such a lot of waiting involved in cancer treatments, but I don't ask people about their disease or the prognosis or the treatment plan. But sometimes they want to talk about it.

Chi'en tells me straightaway. She had breast cancer six years ago, and it has metastasised to her skull and elsewhere. She says softly, 'I am not likely to live another year.' A single tear appears in the corner of her eye; I watch it roll down her cheek. This delightful woman is the only member of her family who is in Australia, apart from her son. She and her husband came to Australia from Taiwan when she was very young, and soon after she had a baby he left her and went back. Chi'en decided to stay in Australia, and has been a single parent ever since.

Her son is the apple of her eye. He is a gifted musician and a PhD candidate in physics. He visits his mother for several hours every day. She beams when she speaks about him, and she loves life and nature. She has no specific religion, but says she believes in a higher power. Every day when I'm leaving, she asks me to pray for her. I say 'OK.' On the way home, I think about what it means, to pray. Simone Weil wrote in *Gravity and Grace* that any undivided attention is prayer. Maybe here it means to say softly to no one in particular, *Let Chi'en get better. Let Chi'en get better.* So I do that. It doesn't work.

Glaring

Jock was admitted late yesterday afternoon, and on my morning round today, I looked in on him, but he was asleep, so I planned to see him tomorrow. We are having lunch when a phone call comes in from Emma, one of the nurses on my ward, asking me to see a patient. The message is that 'the patient is in need of pastoral care'. Most of the afternoon is going to be taken up with case-study presentations, so I ring the ward and speak to Emma. I say Jock was asleep when I was on the ward, and ask if he is awake, and she says, 'Yes … He is …' in a hesitant way that is hard to interpret.

I find Jock sitting on the edge of the bed, his chest concave and bare, with a jacket draped around his shoulders. On his chest is a large, crudely drawn tattoo of a sailing ship distorted by an impressive scar that extends from the top of his chest down to his sternum. There are numerous other 'stick and poke' tattoos on his arms and hands. They are from a time when getting a tattoo had a different meaning.

There is a tube going into his crooked nose. His head is bent forward. He looks uncomfortable and unhappy.

'Hello Jock?'

A narrow, weathered face looks me up and down suspiciously. He looks like a bogan cyborg.

'I'm the pastoral worker on this ward. My name is Johannes. How are you going?'

'Ah … all right, I guess …' he says noncommitally. He scratches himself.

'I'm just here to have a chat and see how you are going.'

'I'm OK. I don't really need anything.'

There is a short silence. He looks at me again. 'It hurts to talk. I don't really feel like talking.'

'We don't have to talk! I can just sit with you for a while, Jock. Would that be OK? If I sit with you?'

'Yeah, I suppose … I'm about to have a shower, though.'

'That's OK.'

I get a chair and sit there with him for a while. I am looking at Jock's face, observing him, looking for an opening. I could ask about his tattoo. *That must have hurt!* I could say. But he said he doesn't feel like talking. He starts coughing, and a large amount of phlegm and slime comes out of him. I reach over and hand him some tissues, and bring the bin closer so he can reach it. He doesn't acknowledge me, but he takes the offered tissues. He recovers himself, but he is obviously in pain.

Emma walks past and Jock asks, 'Have you got a spare pair of pyjamas?'

'I'll go and have a look,' says Emma. 'I'll help you with your shower, too, in a minute, Jock. There's someone in there at the moment.' She points at the shower.

'OK.'

I sit back down. I'm looking at Jock's face. He's not returning my gaze. I'm trying to work out what's going on for him. He looks up. I look at his eyes. His eyes are blue. His face is indescribably sad. We sit there together for about five minutes, neither of us saying anything. Suddenly, he says sharply, 'So do you just go around and sit there, glaring at people, do you?'

He almost spits it out. He is angry. I am more than a little shocked.

'I'm not glaring at you, Jock. I'm just sitting here with you.'

'Well, it's making me uncomfortable ...'

'If you don't want me to be here, I'm happy to go!'

'OK. Good!'

'OK, Jock. All the best. Take care.'

If I had a tail, it would be between my legs. I feel hurt. This is my lunch hour. I was responding to a referral. A referral is gold. For the most part, this work consists of cold calls and follow-ups from previous visits and other pastoral-care staff. Perhaps it's because it *was* a referral that I felt like I had to make a real effort. If I'd had this conversation with him in the course of my normal round, I wouldn't have felt obliged to persist in the way I did.

But why did Emma think Jock needed pastoral care? Just because a nurse says that someone is in need of pastoral care doesn't make it true. What does Emma know about pastoral care anyway? Or maybe she called us because she's in need of pastoral care herself. Maybe she's at her wits' end with Jock. I'm trying to slink back to the office when Emma spots me in the corridor. She is on her way down, and we walk to the lifts together. She asks how I went with Jock, and we chat about him. She tells me how difficult it has been looking after him. She says he's being very grumpy and uncooperative.

Emma has a ring going through a hole in one of her nostrils. She is maybe 21 or 22, and only a year or two out of university—and she's 'had it up to here' with Jock.

'What made you choose a cancer hospital?'

'Umm ... I thought it would be a challenge?' she says.

'You got that right!'

We laugh and go our separate ways. But I'm shaken. I feel ashamed. I am sad. I think long and hard about why Jock felt like I was glaring at him. Maybe I *was* glaring? I remember looking for an opening. He told me he didn't feel like talking! But I didn't listen! So maybe it was because I wasn't present. I wasn't being there for *him*; I was being there for Emma. And now my little ego feels crushed because I failed. And I was not appreciated. And it was my lunch hour!

At the end of the day, I go back up to the ward to say goodbye to Iris. She is going home tomorrow morning. Like Kelly, she may be going home to die, but she's going home, and everyone loves going home. Iris tells me her daughter is going to be there for her, yes, and she is very upbeat.

Walking home tonight, it's not raining. I am so happy to be able to walk. I do little thinking. I am blasting my eardrums to kingdom come with a live recording of King Crimson from 1972, somewhere in the American mid-west. I've been listening to this piece of music for 40 years, and I'm still discovering new bits in it. At the same time, it's like comfort food. I really need it, after Jock and then three hours of case-study presentations in that stuffy room. At least that sickly indoor plant has gone. I wonder where it went. Did someone take it home, or was it put out of its misery?

Followers

This morning, the skies are full of dark clouds, but I decide to walk to the hospital anyway. This is a mistake. I get rained on—but I needed the fresh air. I'm addicted to the walking, the feeling I get from the blood flowing, the lungs moving in harmony with the legs … 1, 2, 3, 4 … and the thinking I can do—or not do.

I'm starting to feel more able to get my head around the complexity and magnitude of the task of pastoral work, and I'm getting to know some of the staff on my ward. The nurse in charge today is Mabel. She is short, and her head is smaller than you expect a person's head to be. She wears thick glasses. She always takes the time to sit down with me when I get to the ward for my morning round, and she goes through the patients one by one in a thick Chinese accent. There are always at least two or three she thinks should be seen by Pastoral Care. I love her for this. Being of use makes me feel much more at home on the ward.

Mabel says I should call in on Chi'en. The gravity of her situation is becoming clear to her. The tumour in her brain has not responded as well to the radiation treatment as the doctors had hoped. We talk about the birds in her garden, which she loves, and how delicate they are. Once upon a time I would have thought, *Why remind her of what she may never have a chance to see or hear again?* But I've changed my tune (as it were). I get her to describe the colours of their feathers and how they move, and the different songs they sing. The delight on her face! My supervisor says, 'We are followers.' Chi'en wanted to remember her garden, and I followed. For a few minutes, I was able to be there with her.

The millions

Today, Eugene says to me proudly, 'I'm a millionaire, you know!' He's already told me this. Perhaps he's forgotten. Or maybe it doesn't matter to him. He just likes saying it. And he likes hearing himself say it. I remember on my very first day on the ward telling him I don't like talking about money. You can waste countless hours talking about money, and in the end it is just numbers on a piece of paper or on a screen and, although there is plenty of hubris amongst the rich, I'm yet to meet anyone who is truly happy solely as a result of all the money they've got. But that was back when I thought it mattered what I was interested in. What matters is that Eugene is dying. I don't say anything. I just look at him with the new neutral-but-friendly face I've been practising, to see if he wants to say anything more.

'Several times over …' he adds.

'And does that make you happy?'

He looks at me a little suspiciously.

'I know, I know. I can't take it with me …' He pauses, and looks out of the window.

'I s'pose my kids will just fritter it all away.'

In all the conversations we've had, he has never once mentioned having any kids.

'How old are your kids?'

'One is 30 this year. The other is 26.'

'And are they all right?'

'They're both as useless as each other,' he says impatiently. 'They've got no idea how hard I've worked for that money.'

'Well, you don't *have* to leave it to them.'

He grins. 'That would be a good one!'

'You could leave it to the hospital! They'd love to have your money.'

'Imagine that,' he laughs. 'What a surprise they'd get. They'd be spewin'!'

I leave Eugene chuckling.

Silence

Andrew was admitted a few days ago.

'Have you met Mr ... um ...' Ariane, one of the social workers on my ward, asks me after a ward meeting, early on a Monday morning. The meeting started late and ran over time. I'm keen to get back to the office for handover, but I'd like to make friends with Ariane. She is one of the few staff on Ward 8 who gives me the time of day. Ariane always looks exhausted, but today she is pale as a ghost and looks as if she is about to pass out.

She is leafing through the pages on her clipboard, '... in ... Bed 5C ...?'

'Hi, Ariane! How are you? I've been off since Thursday, so I haven't had a chance to see him yet.'

She tells me he lives alone in a caravan park. 'He's a bit of a mess,' she says, 'he might benefit from a chat ...'

'OK! I'll see him this morning.'

As it happens, I don't get there until the afternoon. Andrew is seated on a chair, quite literally in a pool of blood. He is wearing a gown. It is covered in blood, fresh blood ...

coagulating blood … dried-up blood. There is blood on his hands. He is bleeding from the mouth. I can see from the ward sheet that he is about my age, but he looks at least 20 years older.

I tell him who I am. He nods. He bleeds.

'Are you OK? Do you want me to call a nurse?'

He shakes his head, and the tube going into his nose shakes in sympathy. Another tube is going into his arm, and there are several other tubes going in and coming out of various parts of him. There is something inside me, a voice—it is only a small voice, but it is quite urgent and loud. It says: *This is too hard. He is too sick. There is no point!*

I ignore the voice. I ask Andrew if I can sit. He motions to a chair in the corner, and I walk over and get it. The voice says: *He looks a bit crazy.*

There is a small whiteboard on his little table. Andrew picks up the marker that lies next to it and writes with a shaky hand, I.C.A.N.T.T.A.L.K., and puts down the pen.

Some part of me wants to say: *What's with the full stops?* But what I say is, 'It's OK.'

It's not OK. Not at all. But I sit down. 'How is it going?' I ask.

He writes, I.T.H.U.R.T.S.

I say, 'Are you managing to keep your spirits up?'

There is silence. Then there is the squeak of the whiteboard marker on the board as he writes. I watch each capital letter being slowly and laboriously formed.

'I.M.N.O.T.G.I.V.I.N.G.U.P.'

'That's the way,' I say.

Smith taught me to say that. His name was Andrew, too, but no one called him that except the headmaster, when he was in trouble. We were both teachers in the same high school. We were in our mid thirties, but we behaved like teenage boys, laughing at people behind their backs and smoking joints on the way home. But he'd been there ten years, and I was just starting. I'd spent the previous decade taking drugs, and making art, and writing bad poetry. He would ask you how you were, and if you said, 'Ah well … hanging in there …' he would say, 'That's the way!' Before long I was saying it, too, and twenty years later I am still saying it.

And now I am here, saying it to a dying man who has lost his ability to speak. I say, 'You are determined?!'

He nods, and it takes him several minutes to write, I.A.M .G.O.I.N.G.T.O.K.E.E.P.F.I.G.H.T.I.N.G.

It begins to dawn on me that the full stops in between each letter are an integral part of the message. I compliment him on his resilience. He manages the beginning of a smile, but you can see that it is painful. He is trembling all over his body. He is all skin and bone.

It is the tail end of what has not been a good day, a disappointing day, on the ward. I have not got any traction with anyone. I had a couple of unfriendly refusals. George, who has recently undergone a radical laryngectomy, manages to growl, 'I don't really feel like discussing the universe with a pastoral worker at the moment. I hope you can understand that.' I mispronounce his surname. He corrects me. I say, 'Fair enough.' But I'm shaken.

I go back to the office for a cup of coffee. Later, I say to my supervisor, 'I should have said: *Well that's a very large topic. Maybe we could start with something smaller.*' And we both laugh heartily. But George was not in a joking mood, and who can blame him? Sometimes I feel like, with some of the angry patients, that it's almost as if they resent me being well. Like years ago, when I thought some old people hated me for being young.

I have wondered why I was assigned to the head, neck, and lung ward. I didn't put it down as one of my preferences after the tour of the hospital on the afternoon of the first day, because they told us some of the patients on 8 were unable to speak.

In my journal I wrote: *how can you have a meaningful relationship with someone who can't talk? i love words. they're all we've got. words are the only reason i am here. language is what it is all about.*

But now I am grateful. I realise that it's a privilege for me to be here, and to be able to, somehow, make some kind of difference to some of the patients—with or without words.

The people who can't talk can still answer a question with their eyes, or a nod, or a shake of the head. And the people who are prepared to give you the time of day will pull out their board or a pad and a pen, and write down what they want to say to you. It's not that they don't have words; they just don't have functional vocal chords, or they no longer have a tongue, or they don't have enough air in their lungs. That's what they should have said about Ward 8.

I am so grateful to Andrew that he took the time and trouble to engage with me, and I tell him so. I say, 'Thanks for talking to me!'

I watch as he writes, Y.O.U.A.R.E.V.E.R.Y.W.E.L.C.O .M.E

The sound of snowflakes

Andrew has the same haunted look I saw in the eyes of the people in the Nazi photographs of Hungarian Jews waiting for selection on the platform at Birkenau in 1944, when I studied the Holocaust.

I studied the Holocaust because my grandmother was a survivor, although she never mentioned it. She must have spent hundreds, or thousands, of hours talking about her experiences living under Nazi occupation—she never grew tired of telling me about it, and I never grew tired of listening. But not once did she mention that, as the child of a Jewish father, she should have gone to register, but didn't. She should have worn a star, but didn't. She looked exactly like the archetypal Jewish woman the Nazis hated—her nose, her eyes, her mouth. Dead giveaways. How did she manage not to get picked up and sent to Mauthausen? Wasn't she afraid? All of these questions I never got to ask her.

But I read all the Holocaust books I could get my hands on—and there are many. For years I would *only* read books about the Holocaust. I couldn't read fiction anymore. I could only read accounts of how people suffered. And I read the accounts of the people who inflicted the suffering. I looked at thousands of photographs. I listened to the testimonies of survivors in Holocaust museums. I wanted to learn about suffering. I wanted to learn how people coped with suffering. I wanted to know how it was possible for human beings to inflict suffering on other human beings.

One winter, while visiting family in The Netherlands, I caught the train to what had been East Berlin. At the old

Ostbahnhoff station, I boarded a train to Poland. In the Ibis Krakow, I asked the receptionist to write 'Return ticket to Auschwitz' in Polish on a piece of paper, and I showed it at the ticket window at the station and handed over 14 zlotys. 'The Museum', as it is referred to by the locals, is only 65 kilometres from Krakow, but it takes nearly two hours by train because it stops at every single one of the bleak and tiny signless snow-covered stations in various states of disrepair on the way. I can see why the bus operators do such a brisk trade, taking tourists there for 140 zlotys.

The train is everything you'd expect from a machine built in the eastern bloc in the sixties. It is the plainest of old rattlers, functional with working heaters, but either thermostats were considered a sign of a bourgeois lifestyle or they're broken. But no matter, with the outside temperature around eleven degrees below zero, when it gets to about 40 inside the train, and the conductor gets around to it, the heaters are switched off—and then, when it drops to zero, they eventually get switched on again.

I get off the train at Oswiecem station and walk the two kilometres to the camp through the thick snow as a kind of pilgrimage, although I am well aware that this is not where they had arrived. Their trains went directly to a specially built platform at Birkenau, another three kilometres away. The irony is that those who made it to the *Arbeit Macht Frei* sign in Auschwitz I were the lucky ones.

Every possible way of killing and humiliating human beings was explored here, and sophisticated systems were developed for doing so en masse. Block 11 is the death block.

In its dark, windowless basement are the 'standing cells', three of them together—cells within a cell. The prisoner was required to crawl into the space, which is about a metre square and a metre-and-a-half high, through a hole on the ground level. Each of the standing cells accommodated four prisoners.

Over there is the processing area for those who were about to be shot. They were made to undress, both to maximise their humiliation and in order for their uniforms to be more efficiently recycled. Then they were led up via a back door and down some steps to the shooting wall. I've brought my camera, but I can't bring myself to take a photograph. There is no way of capturing or interpreting with a camera what it means to be here. But I find myself alone for a few minutes in the only gas chamber at Auschwitz I, a prototype used for testing Zyklon B. Its inbuilt incinerator, consisting of two large ovens side by side, has a capacity of 'only' 700 *stück* at a time. I get out my voice recorder, and press record. I am hoping the machine can hear the snowflakes falling softly outside. Despite the crows' complaining, the silence is deadly.

As a result of studying and thinking about the Holocaust, I've brought to pastoral work the beginning of an understanding of suffering, or at least an insight into it—but it remains sadly inadequate. The testimonies of those who suffered and survived are, on the whole, about suffering in the past. The testimonies we will never hear are the ones from those who died in the forests and in the camps. Although many who survived continue to suffer the effects of the past in the present, I was listening to their memories of suffering, of the suffering of their friends and families, their experience of the ineffable cruelty of other human beings—and it helped me understand what it means to suffer. But as far as making a difference to them, to be of use, in the present, I was superfluous.

And now, I am here, listening to and being with people who are suffering in the present, learning about suffering from Andrew and others. But who is the perpetrator? I suspect that there are patients—I am just waiting for one of them to say something—who think that I represent the omniscient supernatural being who they hold responsible for them having this terrible disease.

After hours

As the duty pastoral worker, you are the only worker on duty for a 24-hour period. You may be asked to provide pastoral care anywhere in the hospital, not just on your own ward, as is the case during the week. You are on call, which means you may be required to come in to the hospital at any time for urgent cases, usually when someone is dying or has died. Some of my most significant encounters take place when I am the duty pastoral worker on weekends.

It's a Saturday. I am on call. Saturday is sausage day at home. Carnivores like to joke about vegetarian sausages, but they are OK, really—you can put sauce on them, and no one has to die.

It's almost 5.00 pm when the phone rings. A voice says, 'Is that the duty pastoral worker?'

'Yes. That's me!'

'This is the switchboard at the hospital. I have a call for you from Ward 5?'

'OK …'

There is a click, and a voice says, 'This is Henrietta on Ward 5 …'

'Hey! Hello, Henri …'

The nurse in charge on 5 today, Henrietta, is known to all and sundry as Henri. If you have to be called back to the hospital on sausage day, when your only access to the world is via Punt Road, and the Magpies have been playing Hawthorn, you'd want it to be by Henri. Cool, but approachable and friendly, respectful, super-efficient and highly intelligent, Henri is my favourite nurse in the hospital. Ryszard is the reason Henri rang me. She says he asked if there was someone he could talk to.

'And you're the only non-medical staff on call,' she says. 'Sorry!'

'Don't be sorry,' I say. 'It's OK. I can be there in twenty minutes, depending on the traffic …'

'Thank you!' She sounds genuinely grateful.

I bore my way through the football traffic in my battered Astra. It takes well over half an hour for a trip that takes less than ten minutes at eight o'clock on a Sunday morning. It is an emergency, but not a medical emergency. I sometimes regret having done a doctorate in philosophy instead of something useful like medicine, or, for that matter podiatry, but not today. This is a matter of life and death, although what I do has no influence on its timing.

When I get to the ward, Henri tells me that Ryszard's wife,

Dorota, is 'actively dying'. I think what that means is *actually* dying. She will be dead soon. Bob Dylan said that you're either busy being born or busy dying, but it seems a cruel irony that for many people, death, like birth, is something that happens *to* them rather than it being something they do.

A slight woman in her early sixties wearing a muddy-brown knitted hat, Dorota worked at the hospital, and everyone seems to know her. On my round that morning, she was fading in and out of consciousness. My report said:

> I spent a bit of time sitting with her and holding her hand. She was unable to speak but she smiled at me and acknowledged my presence. Marja, her daughter was in attendance and she appeared strong and resolved. She expressed the wish that her mother would not have to suffer much longer.

Henri accompanies me to Dorota's room and introduces me to Ryszard. She is much more alert than this morning. There is no sign of Marja or her younger brother. Ryszard tells me that 'the other members of the team' are out having their dinner. I offer to come back a bit later to give the two of them some time together, but Ryszard asks Dorota if she will be OK by herself for a little while, because he wants to talk to me. 'This wreck of a man needs some looking after, too,' he tells her with a weary smile.

Dorota attempts to smile, as if to say that she doesn't object. I touch her arm, and she turns to look at me.

'I'll do my best to help him.' I *think* she heard me.

Ryszard suggests we go into the day room, and we walk

the seemingly deserted ward together in silence. It smells of hospital dinners, and here and there the sound of cutlery on porcelain can be heard. Someone, somewhere, is having a coughing fit. I am thinking about my sausages.

The TV is blaring in the dayroom. On the screen, ecstatic Magpies fans are celebrating their win against the premiers, as only they can. Ryszard looks around for the remote control, finds it, and turns off the TV. I haven't had much to do with patients' families, and I'm not sure what my role is here. As I am considering this, Ryszard says, 'I don't know quite how this process works, but I wanted to speak to someone because … I am just not coping.'

I hear myself saying confidently, 'OK, well, the way it works is that we have a conversation about what is troubling you'—in the same way I might have spoken to a student about his or her artwork.

'I see.'

'So can you tell me what is happening for you?'

He says nothing.

'In what ways do you feel you are not coping?'

He is thinking, it seems. A clock is ticking more loudly than it usually does.

'I keep losing it. The slightest thing will set me off—an object in the house, or when someone rings me up to find out how she is going.'

He weeps.

'Once it is all over, I'll be OK. I'll be able to get on with coping with life without her. But now it's …'

Behind him, in the corner on a shelf, is a tissue box with pictures of frangipani flowers. When I arrived in Australia thirty years ago, I'd never seen, much less smelled, a frangipani, and right there and then the air was thick with their perfume. I grab the box and put it on the table within his reach. He dries his tears.

'It must be very difficult.' That's all I can think of saying.

He starts telling me about his hearing aid. 'It's *very* expensive ... near the top of the range ...' but he suspects it may not be working properly because he can't hear what Dorota is saying. He says her speech is slurred, and he feels useless because he's unable to help her or do anything for her, and since Marja arrived she's completely taken over.

He looks immensely sad now. I feel like I'm marooned on an uninhabited island with this man, and I have no idea how to help him or how to do anything for him. He explains that this is the second marriage for both of them. His children have sided with his ex-wife—and Dorota's children with their late father.

'They seem to think she should have stayed a lonely widow,' he says angrily.

Do people perform anger to dissolve sadness? I wonder to myself.

'Marja doesn't even live in Australia! She comes to visit maybe once every two years, and even then she only stays a week or two. Marja's only brother is younger than her. When his father suffered a fatal heart attack, he took it hard, and blamed Dorota. He hasn't had any contact with his mother for seven years, and then suddenly he shows up yesterday—alerted by Marja, no doubt,' Ryszard scoffs.

'But Ryszard, you can still be with her and tell her that you love her.'

'It's pronounced *Ree-zjard*, not *Rye-zard*.'

'Sorry.'

'It's OK.'

The clock's ticking is now unbearably loud. *Is it really necessary to have a ticking clock where people are dying?*

He tells me Marja sleeps in the room with Dorota, and cares for her around the clock. 'I can't get any time with her!'

It's like a competition!

'Do you normally get on OK with Marja?'

He tells me they've never been particularly close, but Marja was 'trying' for her mother's sake. But since Dorota has been ill, he's noticed that Marja no longer signs her emails 'love Marja', but just 'Marja'. There is also a lot of tension between him and her brother, whose seven-year absence caused Dorota much heartache.

'This is a very difficult time for everyone in the family, and everyone is grieving. No one is getting enough sleep, no one is eating properly, everyone is in a heightened emotional state,' I say.

He nods. He seems lost in thought.

'What you must try and do is cut each other as much slack as possible. Be your most compassionate and most loving self.'

I am thinking about climbing on a chair, taking the clock off the wall, and pulling the battery out.

'Marja is losing her mother. I think she needs to feel that she is doing all she can to make her last days bearable.'

But I am not sure Ryszard wants to hear what I think. I suggest a family meeting. He seems resistant to that. He thinks it will upset Marja and her brother.

Ryszard tells me that he and Dorota have been together for 12 years.

'We were so happy. We loved each other so much. It was the perfect relationship. All our friends remarked on it.'

He looks at me intently.

'We never had a single argument in 12 years. And now this?'

It's as if he is demanding an explanation from me.

'So what I'm hearing is that you wish that you could have had more time together?'

'I promised her that we would stay together for 30 years!'

He weeps again.

'But that's how we live our lives,' I say. 'We live as if we are immortal. That's the only way we *can* live. Your promise was made in the *hope* that you would both live at least another 30 years.'

Ryszard looks at me. He says he's trying to get all the finances sorted before she dies so he can get Dorota's signatures on the appropriate documents to avoid confusion or problems. He's told her children that his and Dorota's wills are identical: both of them are leaving everything to each other. But he's asked Marja and her brother to make a list of everything they want from the house, in terms of their mother's possessions, and they have done that.

He says very formally, 'I've responded to those lists by agreeing to around 80 per cent of the items, but there are items I would like to keep until I die. Then they can have them. Dorota's children have expressed their unhappiness about this. But I feel I am being very reasonable.'

Having regained his composure by talking about money and possessions, he smiles at me in a calm and reassuring way, as if inviting me to agree with him—like a politician.

Ryszard tells me he is writing a eulogy and putting together a slide show of pictures of Dorota for the funeral. When he wrote to Marja asking for pictures of Dorota from before their marriage, he received a less than generous response.

I feel like saying, *Do you think that is necessary to do all this at this time? Wouldn't it be better to …* But what I say is, 'I am hearing that you feel powerless to do anything practical to help the situation, and so you are doing these things in order to feel like you are helping?'

Ryszard agrees. 'I am a very practical man. Engineer by trade. I've always looked after the finances in the household.'

He tells me that he and Dorota were girlfriend and boyfriend when he was twenty and she was fifteen, but the relationship ended and they each got married. After his marriage broke down and she lost her husband, they met again—at the hospital, of all places—when his mother was dying of cancer. Dorota was working here. They've both always been clear that they don't want unnecessary medical treatment, and he hopes that Dorota's life will end soon, because 'this is not a life'. This morning, Marja too had told me she hoped her mother would soon be relieved of her suffering. Despite their differences, they both want the same thing for Dorota. And both of them are probably also looking forward to the end of their own suffering.

Ryszard tells me he doesn't believe in God, but he prays anyway. This is fascinating to me. *Yes. You cannot believe in God, but believe in prayer!* A prayer is an articulation, like a story or a visualisation. It is like asking for a realisation. Or it can be like that.

'That's OK. You can still pray.'

Everyone wants to believe in something. I want to believe in m-theory, one of the theories in quantum physics. M-theory proposes that there are eleven dimensions and ten-to-the-power-of-five-hundred universes, all running in parallel to this one. But only electrons are able to move between them. And yet to me it seems as if, on rare occasions, we get a sense of one of the other universes, like the feeling when you experience *déjà vu*. It's a glimpse ... or glimmer. And sometimes it's almost as if you're presented with an opportunity to sidestep into one of the parallel universes, or we encounter a wormhole and we just fall through it, into an entirely different realm.

I like the word 'realm'. It contains the word 'real', and I believe the realm in which we dwell is culturally determined. It's the result of our understanding of reality and our belief system, and the history of that understanding and belief system. I want to believe that if we change our idea about reality and how it works and what it is, as a result of a realisation, we can find ourselves in a different realm. Isn't this how I entered the realm where I am now—a pastoral worker in a cancer hospital, and not a lecturer at a regional university? And I want to believe that Ryszard could enter a realm where he is a man with unlimited patience, tolerance, and empathy, and I want to invite him to step into that realm. But I'm not sure that I would be able to facilitate the realisation that is required to bring it about. I guess I could pray for a wormhole.

Could I have handled it differently? This was complex, but was it a kind of spiritual crisis? What is spirituality? Oddly, this is a question that is not often addressed by believers.

Everyone assumes it means what they believe it means.

Ryszard needed someone to hear his story, and I'm glad I was able to be there for him and that he felt able to tell it to me. But where does pastoral work begin and end? I guess you could ask where does the material end and the spiritual begin? And at which point does it become an issue for the social work or psychiatric departments?

But I have to admit to an aversion to the word 'spiritual'. Maybe it's because it reminds me of the 'spiritus' my grandmother used to clean the windows with, which happened regular as clockwork every Tuesday. Clean windows were very important to my grandmother. It's a good thing she can't see the windows in my apartment. One day when I was very young, I put my nose close to the open bottle, and the smell was unlike anything I'd ever experienced before. And I certainly never wanted to experience it again.

So maybe we need to reclaim the word 'spirituality'. Spirituality defies definition. The problem of the nature of spirituality cannot be approached using logic or reason. The rational method is not appropriate for the immaterial, and it is not effective. It is the ineffable. You can't say what it is, although you can say what it is not. What you can say is, it is not material. It is not about the body. It is beyond Newtonian physics. All you can do really is to leave a space for what is unsayable and unknowable. And for sausages! I certainly have room for them.

Henri looks up from the screen when I pass the desk on my way out.

'See you, Henri. Thanks for the referral!'

'Sorry to call you out.' She makes a face.

'Not at all. No worries.'

'Did you get anywhere with Ryszard?' She says it like this: *Rye-zard*.

'Yes, I think so. It was good.'

'Thanks so much.'

The traffic has cleared. It will take less than ten minutes to get home. Where is a traffic jam when you need it? I need time to process the events. I am thinking about Ryszard. I too hope that Dorota dies soon, so he can get on with the rest of his life, and Marja can go back to America. I wonder if they'll keep in touch.

Remember to breathe

It's a week later, and I'm late. I'm the duty pastoral worker again, but today is Sunday. I like working on weekends and on other days when normal people have other things to do, like Mothers' Day or the birthday of Christ. My mother is on the other side of the world, and anyway, Mothers' Day was invented by Hallmark.

Christmas Day is my least favourite day of the year. I don't believe in Christ, and I don't believe that turkeys are food. Also, in the southern hemisphere, where I've lived most of my life, it's usually stinking hot at that time of year, and the lights and warm fires that make it so special in the motherland are irrelevant here. It's just not the same gathering around an air conditioner.

Which is not to say I like having to be at work at eight in

the morning, or missing out on a day of rest and relaxation with my loved ones, but I always get up early anyway, and I do some of my best thinking in the liminal time as night becomes day. Maybe this is what makes it difficult to get to work by eight.

Your first job when you get to the hospital is to print out the ward lists. Next, you check to see if there are any referrals from the worker who was on last night, and then you visit each of the wards and ask the nurse in charge if there are any urgent referrals.

I imagine doctors are quite used to it, but for a pastoral work intern it's unusual to walk onto a ward and for the staff to look visibly relieved that you've arrived.

The nurse in charge on 5 today is Louise. She is not from around here. Her accent was forged in the long winters of the Scottish highlands, or in the Gorbals. I have no way to tell the difference.

'Can you please see Kate? She's the daughter of Fred in room 2. He's close to death,' Louise says. 'She's a *wee* bit hysterical!'

The way she enunciates 'hysterical' makes it sound like a disease. Louise gives me an exasperated look.

'OK.'

'… They're in the dayroom,' she motions, and starts walking in that determined way nurses walk.

In the dayroom, Kate is curled up on the couch under a blanket sobbing loudly. A tall, sensible-looking, elderly woman is sitting in a chair by her side, patting her on the back.

'This is Johannes from Pastoral Care,' Louise announces.

She turns on her heel and leaves me to it.

'Hello,' I say.

The elderly woman rises and takes my proffered hand.

'I am Margaret. This is Kate,' she says, pointing at the couch.

I'll be damned if she doesn't have a Scottish accent as well.

'Fred, her father, my brother, is days …'—she hesitates for a moment or two—'or hours … away from dying. But he is not in pain. He is peaceful. And he has said his goodbyes,' she says matter-of-factly.

I nod and smile, and then something makes me move towards the shape on the couch.

'Hello, Kate.' I say softly, 'I'm Johannes from Pastoral Care.'

She raises her head slightly and glances at me through the tears. I drag another chair over and sit down.

'What's happening for you?'

I don't think she is actually able to speak. The sobbing gets louder. I have no idea where this comes from, but I hear myself say, 'Kate I want to tell you something. I lost my father when I was 19. So I know what you're going through.'

This is not strictly true. My father died when I was 19, but I'd lost him a long time before that. And everyone's grief is unique to *them*. No one can truly know what someone else is going through. I remember all those years ago, when he died, being surprised and embarrassed by everyone's concern, and it seemed as if people were expecting me to be a lot more upset than I was. I felt kind of guilty that I wasn't able to be more demonstrative. It certainly wasn't like *this*.

She sits up and says softly, 'You *know*?'

Her face is a mess of red blotches, and strands of blonde

hair are stuck to her cheek, along with dried tears and snot. I reach into the box of tissues on the table behind me and hand some to her.

'Yes.' She blows her nose.

'It was very sudden. I didn't get a chance to say goodbye.'

The sad, brown eyes had cleared somewhat, but now they fill with tears again. She continues to look at me. *Am I helping this situation? I have no idea. But I have to go on …*

'But I talked to him on the phone that morning … I remember …'

My parents were short of money at the time, and the phone was disconnected. My father complained in a letter that he'd been trying to ring me. But my mother expressly forbade me to tell him that the phone had been disconnected because we had no money to pay the bill. I wonder if I still have that letter? When he died, I asked his wife for the letters I'd written to him. He kept all my letters, as I kept all of his, and I still do. He had shown me the little bundle of my letters tied together in a compartment of his small roll-top desk. The most recent of his letters to me were written on a typewriter. I experienced them as impersonal. When I told him I liked handwritten letters, he said, *But my hand writing is illegible!* Which it really wasn't, or it may have been, for people who weren't used to reading it. But now I realise that using a typewriter enabled him to write to me when he was at the office.

She told me he'd been cleaning up just a week or two before he died, and that he had thrown away my letters. She offered me his electric shaver. At home, I opened it up and it was still full of his beard hairs, and the unmistakeable smell of him, the smell of the father. When I was very young he used to let me sit in the toilet with him when he did his morning bowel movement, during which he liked to read the newspaper and smoke a cigarette. I always enjoyed watching how he would fold the toilet paper. He would tear off three pieces and carefully fold each of them over, before arranging them on this leg ready for use.

On the morning of the day he died, I was living in London, and I called him at home on the off chance that he wasn't working. I'd discovered a public phone at the post office which didn't cut you off when your twenty pence ran out, and I used to call him from there. I remember …

Kate begins to sob again.

'Kate, remember to breathe.'

'What did you say?'

'Remember to breathe!'

'Oh.'

There was a long silence, but it was not uncomfortable. It was as if we'd said everything that needed to be said, but neither of us was in hurry to hang up. I remember just listening to him breathe for a minute or two. He died that afternoon. A massive brain haemorrhage, his wife said. They'd been shopping, and when they got home he said, 'I've got a headache. I'm going upstairs to lie down for an hour.' A few hours later, when she went to check on him, she found him dead.

If it had happened now, I would have asked to see the death certificate. I am sorry to say it, but she was a liar, the woman my father left my mother for when I was five. And she was mean. She was my mother's cousin, and my mother tells the story of how she murdered her goldfish with a potato knife when she was little.

I think I was more upset by him throwing out my letters than by his dying. Anyway, I chose not to believe her, and then I hated her even more. We never spoke again. Some months after his death, I heard she had taken up with one of his friends from work.

I rest my hand on the blanket covering Kate's back just between the shoulder blades, and wait for her to breathe out.

With the money he left me, not that it was much, I went and studied acupuncture, and Tai Chi. This is where I learned about breathing.

'Breathe in …' I whisper, 'and breathe out …'

She is doing it.

'Breathe in … breathe out. … It's all right … Breathe in … breathe out. … It will get better. … Keep breathing in … and breathing out … You have to reconnect with your body. … Don't put all your energy into your mind.'

Her crying has stopped. 'Are you still breathing?'

She nods.

'You're still alive!'

Her face is still indescribably sad, but she manages to smile momentarily. She tells me she's worried about what people at school are going to say. I say that most people don't know how to talk about death, and that she can help her friends at school by being empathetic to *them*.

I've spent about an hour with Kate and Aunt Margaret, who has been in the room the entire time. I look over at her and return her smile. I've been grateful for her calm, silent presence.

My pager goes off. It's a message from the Ward Clerk on 4 to ring her. I excuse myself, and go to the front desk to use the phone. She says Jane has passed away. Both daughters and Robert were with her. I met Robert a week ago at a MET call for Jane, his wife. He's a 'firey'. We chatted about fire-fighting. He seemed more optimistic than his wife's condition warranted. But, I thought, maybe he's just an optimistic person. Maybe when you're fighting fires you learn to be a glass-half-full person.

I walk back into the dayroom, and say my goodbyes to Kate and Margaret.

'Remember to breathe …!' I say to Kate.

Jane

I go up to the ward to offer my condolences and to see if there is anything I can do. And then I'm standing in the room with Jane's body, and with Robert and his daughters. Jane's skin is a strange shade of yellow. Her mouth is open. The two women in the room are both crying and looking in disbelief at the body of their mother. She's been dead for maybe half an hour.

The last time I saw a dead person was nearly twenty years ago, when my grandmother died. I refused to view my father's body, despite the urgings. 'It will help you,' they said. 'He doesn't look too bad,' they said. But I wanted to remember him the way he was. But when my grandmother died, I decided I should look. Her face had the expression she wore when she was trying to undo the lid on a jar of pickles.

Robert is calm and dignified. He is drinking a cup of tea.

He holds the saucer with a spoon on it, in one hand, and the cup in the other. He says they are comforted by the fact that they were all able to be there with her until the end, and places the empty cup on the saucer. He is being brave. He has been defeated, but he has known defeat before. Now it seems as if he knew all along that it would end this way, but his duty was to keep hoping, to keep looking for signs that she might recover, not just for himself but for 'his girls.' He did his duty as a husband and a father until the end.

I put my hand on his shoulder. 'I'm sorry.'

He says softly, 'We're OK.'

I don't believe him, but all I can do is believe him. I walk over and take the hand of one of the daughters. I say it again. It's all I can think of. And I am.

'I am so sorry.'

She doesn't so much smile as grimace in acknowledgement. After standing there for a while with them, I say, 'Please call us if there is anything we can do, or if you just need someone to sit with you, or with Jane.' They are all politeness, and attempt to smile to demonstrate their OK-ness.

I am mostly silent for the rest of the day. I am tired. I feel weird. I am full of sadness, but it is a dull, aching sadness rather than a sharp grieving. There is also a sense of wonder and gratitude for having been able to be there for them on this day. But I feel sad about Kate. There is no doubt about that. And I feel sad about Robert (and Jane).

'She's *got* to come back,' Robert had said to me only a week or so ago, when we were discussing Jane's minimal progress.

'I wouldn't know what to do with myself.' We laughed together. Said that way, it was a simple matter.

On my way out, I have a conversation with Raymond and his wife. He has a spark in his eye, despite what he calls 'a seventeen-year battle with cancer'.

'Being in a good relationship can be a big help, can't it?' I say. 'The support can make such a difference.'

He 'couldn't agree more,' and then he looks at his wife with such love and understanding.

At the tram stop, Emma, the friendly nurse from 5, is waiting.

'Didn't Nerida want to talk to you this morning?'

She must have seen Nerida shake her head emphatically when I asked if she felt like a chat. We have a nice exchange about Nerida and how grumpy she gets.

'When are you on next?' I ask.

'I've got three days off!'

'Have you got plans?'

'Vegeing in front of the TV … cleaning the bathroom. You?'

'Tomorrow, 8.45. Ward meeting. The fun never stops!' She smiles, and gets on the 109. I hope the 112 is not far behind.

A universe could form in this room …

New universes are being formed continuously, not with a big bang but in the smallest quietest possible way, according to Sean Carrol, professor of physics at the California Institute of Technology. A universe could form inside this room, and we'd never know. So much for the big-bang theory.

'But *why* are you an atheist?' a Christian asks of me.

'Well, actually, I am an agnostic, but it sounds so wishy-washy.'

They don't say, 'So why are you agnostic?' My response would have been, 'Why are you *not* an agnostic?' But like I said, I think the answer is that everyone wants to believe in *something*.

There are as many possible answers to the question 'What is an agnostic?', which I do get asked regularly, as there are universes. One is: It means that sometimes you do, and sometimes you don't—which is the cute answer. Another is: Believers have their faith, and agnostics have their doubt. I'm still waiting to be asked what I am agnostic *about*. It's always assumed that you're agnostic about God. And although I want to believe, I am agnostic, too, about the ten-to-the-power-of-five-hundred universes and the eleven dimensions, I console myself with the fact that there are some very clever people who can (by a method that I don't for a moment pretend or aim to understand) demonstrate, using mathematics, that the ten-to-the-power-of-five-hundred universes and eleven dimensions are the only way of explaining what exists. I think the existence of God is not impossible either, but I've heard of no one who can demonstrate that omnipotent supernatural beings exist rationally, although a few have tried.

I do appreciate the many uses of reason. I live as rationally as possible. It seems the best way available of working out how to organise things in our society—which is not to say that we *are* doing that—and how to get things done, from the grocery shopping to going to the moon. But is it also the best way to think about the meaning of our lives? *Cogito ergo sum* is the biggest furphy the human race has ever been sold, or maybe free-market capitalism is, but if so it runs a close second. When people ask what I believe, some days I'll say I'm an atheist, and other days I'll say I'm an agnostic. Sometimes I respond by saying that some days I'm an atheist and other days I'm an agnostic. Maybe it would be better to think in terms of what you *want* to believe, or what you *don't* want to believe. What I don't want to believe is that we live in a cold, dark, rational universe where everything we experience as true and beautiful is just the result of an accidental encounter between two or more of the ingredients of a cosmic soup.

'You just have to believe,' a priest told me when I was a teenager teetering on the edge. 'Or it wouldn't be called a faith.' He was the Reverend Jim Thompson, who later became the Bishop of Stepney and a regular contributor to *Thought for the Day* on BBC4. He died suddenly on a cruise ship off the coast of Spain in 2003, in the middle of a sermon, a bit like Tommy Cooper. *Just like that.*

Speaking of faith, although I am a non-believer, I'm open-minded. Is that faith? But my faith is an ever-evolving faith, and my doubt is always there right alongside it. What I believe is changing, growing, reducing, expanding—as information becomes available, and as I experience the world and all the things in it, and as I think of things—in short, as I live my life, and as I, hopefully, become better at being a human.

But, of course, all of this probably precludes me from being a 'real' atheist. I don't think the Australian Atheist Association would have me as a member. I am not dogmatic enough. I am more interested in opening doors than closing them.

During my year as an agnostic pastoral worker I had a lot to do with Christians who are frightened or depressed by atheists, so I prefer to say: 'I am a non-believer. I don't believe in a god, but I don't believe in atheism either.' And if you ever need to get a group of Christians on side, this is what you should say. Then, when the laughter dies down, you can become more serious and you can talk about what you do believe in.

I also advise that, when talking to Christians, you let it be known that some of your best friends are Christians and that you don't believe any atheist should be telling anyone that they shouldn't believe what they want to believe. But, by the same token, I don't believe Christians should be trying to convert people to believe what they believe, and frightening small children by telling them that they will spend eternity burning in hell.

I also think that what you believe is the most important thing in the universe, or at least in this particular universe — because what you believe, or don't believe, informs your actions.

In terms of my work in the hospital, I'd envisaged that I would be a pastoral worker for atheists, but that's not how it's working out. A pastoral worker has to be able to work with anyone, regardless of their belief or disbelief. Nevertheless, I especially wanted to be there for the non-believers, particularly those who had dedicated their lives to eliminating from their consciousness the slightest inkling or idea about transcendence, or the possibility of anything existing that is not material — those who remain unwilling to the very end to believe in an afterlife where a supernatural omnipotent daddy can make everything all right. They are anti-immaterialists. They are in denial about the possibility that some things (for the want of a better word) cannot be nailed down by reason, common sense, and Newtonian physics. There is plenty of evidence—good, rational, scientific evidence—for the immaterial, as we discover when we enter the realm of quantum theory. But let's not go there. It is endless, and, since it has no beginning either, you're already there. And so am I.

I am here.

Marjorie

I wanted to be there for Marjorie, but she didn't want me to be there, not until the very end. And I never had the opportunity to have this discussion with her—or, for that matter, any other discussion of significance. If I introduce myself to a person in the hospital as a pastoral worker and they say 'I'm not a Christian,' it gives me the opportunity to tell them I'm not a Christian either—and an interesting conversation can follow. And if my own beliefs come up, as they sometimes do, I'm *in*—because I am happy to talk about what I believe, or about what I believe is possible—which is everything.

And this creates an opportunity for people to talk about *their* beliefs. And to any Christian who is at all concerned that I don't believe in God, I'll use the 'Some of my best friends are Christians!' line. I also have best friends who are atheists, but there is no need to mention that. There are also plenty of people who say, 'I'm OK, thank you' when I introduce myself, and who don't stop reading their book and/or looking at the TV or their computer screen. What do you say to that? That was Marjorie.

One day, when I have come to see someone else in her room, I say to Marjorie, 'Nice computer!' She is using a Macbook Air. People who use Apple products usually enjoy hearing you say that you like their computer. Or they used to. Marjorie looks up, as you might at an annoying child.

'Yes, yes.'

'Do you have internet in here?'

'Yes.' She points at the wireless USB modem sticking out the side, and she goes back to what she was doing.

I want to say: *If you have any problems with your computer … my other job is in computer support. Give me a call!* But I'm not that desperate—although, later, on the last day of her life, I did end up helping her with an audio-visual problem.

Back in the office, I write in my journal:

> marjorie says she is fine but i am not convinced. she doesn't seem interested in talking and the visitor she had with her today, eyed me suspiciously when i came into the room. try again?

I wouldn't go so far as to say my relationship with Marjorie was immaterial, but it certainly lacked substance. My interactions with her were so short that they remained mostly undocumented. It's not really worth recording in the ancient record-keeping system, which is still in use at the hospital, designed in the early nineties by an IT guy with a peculiar sense of humour, that you said hello to someone and they said hello back in such as way as to make it very clear that they don't want the conversation to go any further. Each kind of pastoral encounter is supposed to have a two-digit code, but there is no code for that.

Marjorie was in a room with other patients during most of her time in the hospital, which was a long time — many months. I'd always give her a friendly wave, or say hello in passing, and sometimes I would stop and ask her how she was going. She was never impolite, but her politeness was the kind that middle-class people use in lieu of rudeness. And yet I did have a relationship with her. She knew who I was, and she would always return my greeting, no matter how tersely.

Almost every ward meeting I attended during Marjorie's stay in the hospital would end with the nurse in charge saying something despairing, like, 'Marjorie is in denial. She wants to go home.' And the physio might say, 'She can't even manage the four steps she would have to negotiate there.' And one day someone said, 'She says her boss is holding her job open for her until she gets back.' I'm sure I could see her rolling her eyes. But was Marjorie a fool for thinking or hoping or believing that she would recover?

For the medical staff, Marjorie was being 'unrealistic'. She was 'in denial' about the seriousness of her disease. She was being 'irrational'. But reason and rational thought are not necessarily the tools that people will choose when they are trying to deal with the fact that they have a terminal illness and that they're going to die.

And I am the one person on that team who will not throw up their hands in despair if you say you're going OK on the day you die. If you believe right up to your last laboured breath that you're *not* dying, and that you *are* going to get well again, then I am OK with that. I am here for you to talk about what it means to be dying, but only if you want to talk about it, if you want to think about it. If you choose not to, if you choose not to believe it, it is your life. Who am I to question that? And that was Marjorie on the last day of her life.

'How are you, Marjorie?'

'I've had a rough couple of days. But I'm coming right now.'

I was the duty pastoral worker on the day she died. The charge nurse had told me she was deteriorating, so I called in to see her. Marjorie was very uncomfortable with her breathing, and just generally. She'd been moved into a single room. I thought, *Perhaps the end is nigh for her.* It was the first time I'd ever seen her by herself, and she was more forthcoming than she had ever been, not that that's saying much. She asked me to turn on the TV. Never before had I been able to do anything at all for her. I turned on the TV and gave her the remote control. I stayed for a while in silence, thinking about the fact that I'd made some progress in my pastoral relationship with her. Then she suddenly said, 'If you don't mind, I'd like to rest now, thank you.'

'OK!'

I wished her all the best, and then I was gone. Back in the office, I wrote:

> Some people just believe that they are going to get better despite all the evidence to the contrary. I guess she will die at some point in the middle of believing that, and who am I to say that she should think anything else. Just

because you're dying doesn't mean you want to think about death, just like the people who are living who don't want to think about life.

At five o'clock I received a call from her nurse, Carly. Marjorie had died around 4.00 pm. I was stunned. I was expecting it, but not today. I guess she was not expecting it either, or maybe she was. Who knows?

I go to the hospital and offer my condolences to the family, who are present at the bedside — two brothers, the wife of one of the brothers, and Marjorie's young niece. They are all quite composed and relieved. Marjorie's suffering is over.

'She is at peace.'

One of the brothers explains that she is with their younger brother now. He died twenty-two years ago yesterday. The brothers spend some time remembering Marjorie, and sharing stories about the good times they'd had together. They all thank me for being there. Then they ask me what happens from here. I was not expecting that. I have absolutely no idea. I promise to come back soon. I go back to the office. I remember seeing a leaflet there with *When a Patient Dies* on the front. I read it, and go back down to explain the procedure.

The hospital doesn't have a mortuary. It has an arrangement with a funeral home. They store the body. The brothers want to take Marjorie's phone. They also want to know if they can take her watch and glasses, which she is still wearing. I go and get Carly. She thanks me for coming and says, 'They can take her phone. And they can take her watch and glasses off, too, if they want, or we can do it for them.'

I go back in and tell the brothers what Carly said. Everyone is nodding, but no one makes a move towards Marjorie, or her watch, or her glasses. I shake all of their hands, and briefly touch Marjorie's arm by way of saying goodbye.

This was one of the least satisfying pastoral relationships I've had at this stage of my fledgling career, but I've done everything I could for her—that is, if all you can do is what people will allow you to do. And until I turned on the TV for her this morning, she had never allowed me to do anything for her. I never knew anything about her, except her age. She was exactly the same age as me. I never read her medical notes. Her brother said she'd never married and never had any children. Did she have any friends? I wasn't game to ask. I never saw anyone visit. She was so stand-offish; she was intensely private. She died alone with the TV on, and death appeared to come easily to her. The remote was still where she'd put it after I'd handed it to her, but someone had turned the TV off. The only mourners were her siblings.

I said, 'She was very independent,' and everyone agreed.

It might seem strange, but I'm glad I was able to have a moment with her on the last day of her life, minimal as it was, and that I was able to be there for her family after her death.

Goodbye to James

James appeared on one of the ward lists this morning. This is not usually a good sign. You'd rather patients didn't come back, because while they're away you can choose to believe they're still in remission. But James was discharged to a hospice, so I didn't think I would ever see him again.

He is not on my ward, but I check with the colleague whose ward it is, and ask if he minds. That's the protocol. We can't have workers randomly going to other people's wards. I'll call in on James before going to my own ward. I am looking forward to seeing him.

The door is closed, and when I knock, a woman about my age, looking somewhat dishevelled and/or underslept, comes to the door and asks me in an irritated voice who I am. This is understandable. There are so many comings and goings here. Is this the daughter who lives in Sydney? I've never met her, and James rarely spoke about her, although I remember she rang once when I was with him and his voice became tender as he spoke to her.

'I am a pastoral worker.'

She seems hostile. I'm not sure if it is my imagination, but it is as if she only just manages to stifle a sneer. She doesn't stop me coming in, though, and I walk to the edge of the bed. James is unconscious. He has lost a lot of weight. His skin is sallow and dried out. I want to say, *I knew him well.* But that would be absurd. I didn't. I try to think of a way to describe our relationship to someone who probably thinks of me as a god-botherer. *We were friends,* I want to say. But that would be overstating it.

'My name is Johannes.'

She says nothing. In her hand is a tube of Sorbolene.

She says, 'I hope you don't mind if I continue?'

'Of course.'

He seems comfortable. I put my hand in his hand. It is

stone cold. But he is still breathing, just. There are long pauses between the breaths.

'Hello, James! Hello, mate.'

No response.

I can see that James is finally ready to die. I am not needed here.

'Bye, James.'

I say goodbye to his daughter, but she is fully absorbed in her work. I close the door quietly behind me. There are tears in there somewhere, but they stay down, more or less.

The next day, he is gone.

My father was not a poet

There are worse things than dying. One is disappearing. One day you're just not there anymore, and no one knows why or where you've gone. In one sense, disappearing is exactly the same as dying: someone is no longer there, but there's no cold, hard body, or no warm, soft body gradually becoming cold and hard as you're standing there with clammy hands clasped behind your back, and a heavy chest.

When someone disappears, something else remains: the *possibility* that they might reappear. There is no solid Nothing, and there is no closure.

When someone dies, you don't know where they are either, but you know what happened. Everyone knows. It's a well-known narrative. If someone asks, you say: 'They died,' and people look concerned and they are nice to you.

I lost my father twice. First, he disappeared. I was five. I couldn't understand why he was gone, or where he went. I simply expected him to come back. I don't really remember anything but a vague sense that one day he would just be there again, like he always was before. I don't remember him saying goodbye or explaining why he was leaving. If he'd been a poet, maybe he would have written a poem about it, and I could read it now, but he was a policeman. My mother must have tried to explain it to me, but I don't remember the explanation. Or maybe she was too devastated herself to understand it, let alone explain it to a five-year-old.

There is a gap in my memory, too, an absence. I have plenty of memories from before, but then ... nothing, for a long time, a year or more. I don't remember moving house. I don't remember my first day at school. I do remember crying a lot in my first years of school. I would cry at the drop of a hat.

And he wasn't there for a long time, and then he periodically reappeared, usually to argue with my mother about money and make her cry—or she made him cry and stamp his foot—and then he disappeared again, and I got used to the comings and goings.

And then he died. But that was later. And, in a way, that made it better. Being dead is something everyone can understand.

Julia

Qualifications

It is winter. I am a qualified pastoral worker—or, to be more accurate, I am in possession of a piece of paper that says I've achieved a basic level of competence as a pastoral-care practitioner. This is no less astonishing to me than when I was given a piece of paper by a real university, albeit one in the middle of nowhere with a name which means 'place of many crows', which told the world that I was a doctor—not a doctor of something practical or lucrative like medicine, but of philosophy, which should be the most important thing in the world, but isn't. As soon as I learned that there were philosophers, that there were people whose *job* it was to think about the meaning of life—which has puzzled me since I learnt the meaning of 'meaning'—I wanted to meet one and, when I was thirteen, I did. The father of my stepfather's brother-in-law was introduced to me as a philosopher, and now I wonder if I was the butt of a practical joke. But I took it very seriously.

As a child, I always believed everything people told me. It didn't occur to me that anyone would say anything that was untrue. Why would they? My father thought this was hilarious. He told me that you could frighten monsters and make them go away by yelling 'Poo!' at them. Actually, that may be true. But he also told me chewing gum was made from old bicycle tyres, and this non-fact lodged itself in a corner of my brain for thirty-five years. One day, I was walking along thinking about chewing gum when I suddenly thought, *Hey! That is absurd! It can't be made from old bicycle tyres!* And I remembered how heartily my father would have laughed if he had known it would take me the best part of forty years to work that out. But I guess it was stored in a part of my brain that I didn't access during that time. Why would you think about what chewing gum is made of?

The philosopher was Italian and didn't speak a word of English, and at the time my command of that language was not much more than rudimentary. The brother-in-law acted, somewhat half-heartedly and all too briefly, as translator. Gesturing and sign language don't really cut it when you're trying to discuss the meaning of life. The philosopher smiled a lot, and pointed at the sky, and said some things in Italian. He was old and grey and wearing a nice suit. I was sure he knew the answer to the meaning of life, but I couldn't get it out of him in an intelligible form. I went away disappointed, but I liked his aura.

I received my certificate on the day I met Julia. She, much more than the piece of paper, eventually persuaded me that I was qualified as a pastoral worker. The fact that it was on this day that I first met her became very significant to me. We say 'that was meant to happen' about events later, with the benefit of hindsight, but never before it happens. Or we say it, and then it doesn't. Sometimes we say 'Everything happens for a reason' because that makes for a better story—but here we are gesturing at an intuitive feeling that there must be things which are beyond reason. Some rational minds are prepared to admit it, and others aren't. Because I am, I guess that makes me an agnostic. Everything is possible.

Jung coined a term to describe the feeling we have when significant events occur simultaneously and we feel that they are connected somehow: synchronicity. But there is no rational explanation for it, and we don't understand how or why it is so. What I think Jung is asking of us, is to allow our minds to accommodate the possibility of the interconnectedness of things beyond cause and effect, beyond reason.

Julia

When I get to the hospital that morning—it is one of those blustery, dark Melbourne mornings when it looks like it could bucket down with rain any moment, but doesn't—there is a referral waiting for me. It is from one of my least favourite nurses on the ward, Justine. The problem with Justine is two-fold: she has a tic, and she doesn't make eye contact when she's talking to you. Rationally, I know it's not her fault, but there is something disconcerting about having a conversation with a person who appears to be addressing someone who is standing slightly to the side and behind you. And when her face twitches, you experience the dual discomfort of looking intently at her whilst feeling the urge to check whether there is, in fact, a person standing behind you and slightly to the side.

When I get to the ward, Justine is glad to see me. She has a whining voice that makes everything sound like a complaint, and at the same time it's as if the words are tumbling out of her. That's the other problem with Justine. But perhaps she's trying to get the words out before she's overcome by twitches.

'So Julia is post-op and she … she is actually ready to go home, but she doesn't want to go. She says she's not ready. She …'

Justine twitches.

'… doesn't feel well. She has no energy. But she needs to eat something. She won't eat. And she needs to get out of the bed and walk around, but she says …'

Twitch.

'… she doesn't feel strong enough. We suspect she might be depressed, and we've had psych in, but she doesn't want to talk to them.'

I am focussing on my breathing. It will be over soon. She is looking intently at whoever is standing slightly to the side and behind me.

'You are the last resort …'

I don't know if it's good or bad to be the last resort.

'I'll see what I can do.'

Justine leads the way. She can be no more than five foot three, maybe four, and I'd be surprised if she weighs fifty kilos. It never ceases to amaze me what some of the nurses can accomplish with the slightest of physical means, and now that I am writing this, I think *How can I say that Justine is one of my least favourite nurses?* She makes me uncomfortable—that's all, really. But that's *my* problem. And there is no doubt that she really cares. She cares enough about her patient to call a pastoral worker if she runs out of ideas. She walks the way some nurses walk. She wears sensible shoes, and you get the feeling that nothing would be able stop her.

I dated a nurse, Verity, when I was in my late teens. She was several years older than me, and truly beautiful. I was smitten. Several weeks before my birthday, she asked for a list of all the Jimi Hendrix records I didn't own — at that time, there would have been about twelve. On my birthday, she handed me a big box containing all of them, as well as a copy of Michael Chapman's *Fully Qualified Survivor*, which was one of her own favourite records. Forty years later, I still play *Fully Qualified Survivor* sometimes, but I rarely listen to Jimi Hendrix.

Justine pauses before we enter room 4.

'She's *fine*,' Justine whispers in the corridor. 'But she doesn't want to go home.' When there is no volume, there is no whine.

'She feels safe here maybe?' I venture. 'How long will she continue to need oxygen?'

'When we try to reduce her oxygen, she complains.' Justine sighs.

On one of my rounds a day or two ago, I had noticed the slight shape attached to various tubes in the bed near the window in room 8 of my ward, but it was immobile, having just come onto the ward after surgery. A scrawled note next to her name on my ward list reads *out of it* and *maybe later?*

'This is Johannes, the pastoral worker I was telling you about, Julia,' Justine says in a firm, clear voice to the shape, from which a head covered with a multi-coloured beanie emerges, blinking.

'What is your religion?' The voice is croaky and English.

'Um … I don't have one,' I say, with some trepidation.

'Thank God. Neither do I,' Julia says.

We are both relieved.

'Umm … I'll leave you to it …' Justine says quietly as she disappears with a nervous smile.

The ward is silent, apart from various monitors bleeping and beeping reassuringly, and the sound of oxygen rushing out of the wall into a tube and then into a person's nose on its way to the lungs. I am wondering what would happen if the oxygen stopped. If there's a power outage, the hospital's generators kick in. They work. I know this because they test them once a week, with a boom, and half the ground floor reverberates. But how long could they keep going? And what if they fail? Is there a backup generator? And a backup for the backup? I can think of no worse way to die than suffocating. I've seen them in the last stages of emphysema, I've seen them on 100 per cent oxygen, when it's not enough because the lungs just don't have the capacity to absorb the oxygen. I've looked into their pleading eyes, and all you can say is, 'I'm sorry', and you are truly sorry with every fibre in your body, and then when you're walking outside after your shift, each breath of the fresh sweet air is precious—even walking up Punt Hill, where a not-insignificant proportion of what enters your lungs is exhaust fumes—and you thank the non-existent gods that you don't believe in that it's not you lying there.

Neither of us is saying anything, but it's not an uncomfortable silence. I'd like to sit down, but I've adopted the practice, if the person I'm seeing is well enough, to wait until they invite me to sit. This is not about manners per se, but out of respect for someone's personal space, of which there is precious little in a hospital.

A tired, thin, drawn face is looking at me intently with blue … no, green-blue … eyes.

'How are you?' Julia asks.

This was about the last question I was expecting. It's rare to be asked how you are by a patient. It is evident you must be better than them, since you're walking around and you're at work.

'I'm good!'

'When the nurse told me a pastoral worker would be coming,' she says, 'I expected a religious person.'

'Well, the hospital recognises that the 30 per cent of patients who tick the 'No Religion' box on their admission form need pastoral care, too. So you could say I am the token atheist in the pastoral-care department,' I say, smiling.

If the truth be known—and who can say if it is or it isn't—I am actually more of an incognito atheist, and I am not sure that this actually reflects the hospital's position, but it ought to, and I wish it did.

She returns my smile.

'That's good.'

Five minutes in, and this is already the most unusual pastoral encounter I've had in my three months in the hospital.

'Do you want to sit down?' Julia asks.

'Thank you.'

'So what does a non-religious pastoral worker do?'

I've had many a meta-conversation about secular pastoral practice, but not with patients.

'Well, I think what I do is not that different from what the religious ones do. In any case, we are taught in our training not to talk with patients about religion, unless they raise it first.'

'OK … How long is the training?'

'I'm doing the full-time internship.'

'I see. So you're an intern.'

'Yes.'

'OK.' She looks thoughtful.

'So we talk to people about what it means for them to be in this hospital, to be diagnosed with this disease …'

I'm leading up to the inevitable question, but Julia says, 'You sound English … but your name is not English.'

'You sound English, too!'

'I came out when I was twelve with my parents.'

'My parents moved to England from The Netherlands when I was fourteen.'

'Ah. That explains it. And then … they came out here?'

'Ah, no … I came out by myself when I was twenty-two.'

'Oh. What for?'

'A woman … and I knew lots of Australians in London. They were always saying, "You should go!"'

'Ah.'

'What was it like for you, as a young person, to move countries?'

'It was awful …' she says with conviction. There's a way of saying 'awful' with an English accent that makes it especially poignant.

'I hated it,' she continues, 'You?'

'The same. England in 1972 was … bleak, especially for a

fourteen-year-old. I had to wear a school uniform! And when I was caught smoking, they were going to give me the cane! My mother was outraged. She threatened them with legal action. I mean ... I'd come from what was then one of the most liberal and progressive countries in the world. Kids only got in trouble for smoking in the classroom. Only teachers were allowed to do that ...' I laugh.

She smiles. She is listening carefully and intently.

Silence again.

'I loved Australia, though, when I came in 1980,' I offer. 'It still felt like the Lucky Country ...'

'Lucky for some!' Julia scoffs.

'Indeed.'

We've made a connection, and it's not just our lack of religion, or what I suspect is our mutual left-of-centre politics, that we have in common. Undergoing something traumatic at a young age — like moving countries — irrevocably changes a person. It marks you for life, and I often connect easily with immigrants. We are all here because, for the most part, we decided to come here. And we miss our motherland, but we couldn't live there any more. It has changed so much, and we ourselves have changed.

One of my colleagues at the university was secretly enrolled in a law degree part time for seven years whilst at the same time holding down a full-time position as a senior lecturer. After completing his degree he walked in to the dean's office on a Friday and handed in his resignation, effective immediately. On the following Monday, he started work as a lawyer at a local firm. Who says you can't keep a secret in a country town?

I couldn't have pulled that off, but I kept sane in my last year as a lecturer at university by training part time as a reality therapist. Reality therapy was all the rage in the eighties, but has since fallen out of favour and been replaced by less idiosyncratic cognitive-behavioural approaches. But I didn't care. I was so full of loathing for the kind of unreality being perpetrated by the university system, and by the unrealistic expectations the bean counters who had taken over the running of it had of the staff, that the idea of being a reality therapist appealed to me. I loved my teacher Maggie, a sprightly Scot in her seventies, and a real 'people person'. She taught me how to listen to what people were *actually* saying, I mean *really* listen, instead of hearing what you believe they are saying. And how to ask questions. The question you need to ask next, Maggie taught me, comes from what they are telling you *now*. And this was invaluable when I was working with people in the hospital, and it remains so in the work I do now.

As in most other psychotherapies, 'personal disclosure' is especially frowned upon in reality therapy. As a pastoral worker, too, I rarely volunteered personal information, but if I was asked, I always happily answered questions about myself, and this is integral in the work of a narrative therapist. Your stories are how people get a sense of who you are and whether they can trust you with *their* stories. This is how people have been connecting with each other since they lived in caves.

Back in room 8 of my ward, Julia sighs. 'I'm so tired. I can't believe how tired I am!' she says.

'That's understandable. You've just been through major surgery!'

'Yes, but I'm just not coping.'

'Well … if you've got no energy, that's not surprising either. It takes energy to cope!'

'And they say I'm depressed …'

'And what do you think?'

She answers my question with a question.

'Do *you* think I'm depressed?'

'I'm a doctor of philosophy, not psychiatry … so I …'

'Oh? You've got a PhD? What in?'

'Fine arts.'

'I always wanted to do a PhD. I started a Masters … but I didn't finish.'

'It's hard to finish things!'

'It's just that I was … I was working full time and trying to do it. I never had time to …'

'Yeah. I did my PhD whilst working full time, and I don't recommend it. But I was working at a university, so, at least in theory, they were supportive of me taking time to do the work I had to do for it.'

'Were you … lecturing …?'

'Yep. In arts practice.'

She sighs again. 'I've always loved art … and design.'

Julia looks very tired. I think maybe I've done enough for now, and I'm about to suggest that she should rest, when she suddenly says, 'Could you … could you hold my hand?'

'OK …' I am hesitant. It's an unusual request.

'It's just that I … I'm just … I just need some human contact, some warmth. You know?'

'Of course.'

I take her thin, small hand in mine. It is very cold. We sit together in silence for a while. The machine next to the bed starts beeping more loudly and rapidly. We've disturbed its connection to the vein in her arm.

'I'm feeling so alone.' She has to raise her voice. 'No one is listening to me. They just want me out of here and out of their hair. And everyone says I only have myself to blame because I'm not eating and I don't have the energy to get out of bed. Even going to the toilet exhausts me.'

A nurse arrives to check the machine. It is not Justine.

'Can we have some privacy, please?' Julia says impatiently to the nurse.

'I just need to check your line there … um …' She is looking at the chart. '… Julia.' The nurse fiddles with the line, and the machine resumes its more reassuring bleeps. Julia looks cross. The nurse is gone. My arm is uncomfortable now, and I want my hand back.

She tells me that she feels like she is coming to the end of her life and that she has an eleven-year-old daughter, Daisy. She plays the piano and loves animals. Daisy wants to be a vet, but she might not get the marks for that.

'Does she understand what's happening …?'

'No … well, she knows I'm sick. Obviously.'

'But she understands it's possible that you're going to die?'

The sound that comes out of her then is a sob, not a word. But I know that it means 'no'.

'We don't know how to tell her. We're talking about it.'

'This is you and …'

'Tom, my partner … her father.'

She weeps. I look around for tissues. There are none. I'm annoyed that I'm thinking about tissues when somebody is telling me something so completely heartbreaking.

'Do you need a tissue? I could go and ...'

'It's OK,' she says. She takes her hand out of mine, and uses it to pull a tiny hanky out of her sleeve. She blows her nose.

'Anyway ...' she says, recovering herself. 'It is what it is.'

'Yes.'

Ceremony

Clinical pastoral education graduation ceremonies are taken very seriously in the hospital, and since they take place during normal working hours, cannot be avoided. There is no box you can tick that says 'Please send me my certificate in the mail'—which has always been my preferred option when I've graduated. Still, the ceremony is planned entirely by the graduands, so you only have to make it as painful as you want, or as your fellow graduands want. People do all sorts of things with fake noses and music and balloons, but the three of us who were left standing at the end of the first unit easily agreed on a very low-key ceremony.

The connection I made in the space of not much more than an hour with Julia left a deep impression. As I am standing there, listening to the speeches, her heartbreaking story is ringing in my ears, and I can still feel her cold, thin hand in mine.

When I was leaving, she'd said, 'I'm really sorry to have taken up so much of your time ...' and I was so moved by her humanity, her integrity. I took her hand again, looked into her eyes, and said, 'Hey! It's OK. That's what we're here for! And I'll be back. OK?'

I hadn't expected any kind of emotion in response to the ceremony but, combined with the events of the morning, and the idea that after this I will actually be qualified, however minimally, to do this work, I choke up when it is my turn to speak. I just keep talking as best I can. And everyone in a cancer hospital is used to tears, especially in pastoral care.

And then it's time for lunch. That's the tradition on graduation days: we don't go overboard, but we celebrate in style. Since I don't drink, I won't smell of alcohol afterwards, so I volunteer to do the on-call shift that night. This means I will do a last round of the wards and follow up any referrals whilst everyone else pretends to do some paperwork for an hour before going home.

I rarely miss drinking. The story I tell now is that I lost so many brain cells to alcohol and drugs that I need every single remaining one of them to be firing, in order to able to function. The truth is, being clear-headed at all hours of the day and into the evening is still a novelty, even after all these years on the wagon. And I certainly don't miss that woozy, boozy, headachy feeling as the alcohol starts wearing off. There is only one cure for that, and that's just deferring the inevitable.

When I return to Julia's room, she is sitting in the chair by the bed, wearing glasses and reading a book. When she sees me, she smiles warmly.

'I don't know what you did this morning, but I feel like I've turned a corner.'

I consider saying, 'I didn't do anything, you did it yourself,' but this is not what she needs right now. She feels that what I did made a difference, and perhaps it did.

'I was just *there* for you.'

She nods. I have no qualms about taking her hand and giving it a little squeeze. She squeezes back. We sit in silence together for a while. It's comfortable.

'I have to go. I've got a few more people to see.'

She asks me to check in on her in the morning, which I say I will gladly do.

Julia's stay in the hospital turns out to be a long one—much longer than the average admission. She is there for almost three months, with a break of a few weeks in the middle. Some people are keen as mustard to leave the hospital, whilst others are extremely reluctant. For Julia, it is where she feels secure—and perhaps you can choose to believe there is a possibility that something can still be done for you if you're in the hospital. A cancer hospital is unique in that respect. Many people are discharged because all that can be done for them has been done, and then it's just a case of making them as comfortable as possible, maybe giving them a bit more time, whilst waiting for the inevitable. The aim is to get people discharged before they begin 'actively dying'.

'No one is dying,' my supervisor said, stroking his beard, in our weekly supervision session. 'People live, and then they die.'

Yes. But. Well, actually, I'm with Heidegger. We are, each one of us, dying continuously from the moment we're born, and we spend most of the time trying to forget about the fact. What we should be doing is meditating each day on the fact of our finitude, like the Japanese samurai. But it's still a useful observation, especially when you are in a cancer hospital and all you can think about is dying. And this is why each day the pastoral-care department eats lunch together and we talk about mundane things, like how often we change our underwear. Some of us, me included, make the most tasteless jokes imaginable, especially at the expense of people who suggest that underpants can be worn a second time if you turn them inside out.

An atheist in a foxhole

My grandmother believed in ghosts, but she was a committed atheist for most of her adult life. She reserved a special kind of pitying laugh for my grandfather and me when we went to church. But, to everyone's surprise, in her latter years she was frequently found with a rosary in her hands. This was when she was infirm and depressed by her powerlessness in the old people's home where her life ended on the very day I returned to the motherland after a seven-year absence.

They say there are no atheists in a foxhole, but I met plenty of them on the wards of the hospital — and if a specialist cancer hospital is not a foxhole, I don't know what is. True nihilists are rare there. You need to believe in something, even if that something is most unlikely — for instance, the idea that the Bulldogs will one day win another flag.

But I wouldn't know if there *were* any nihilists in the foxhole, because a true nihilist is not going to be interested in talking to a pastoral worker, are they? I might as well be wearing a sign around my neck saying *I believe in something*, even if all I truly believe in is that it's important to think about what it means to be a human being and that we talk to each other about it.

Take Derek. I'd doubt that Derek would even think of himself as a nihilist, since most nihilists probably don't believe in being self-reflective either. My encounter with him came in the days following my first couple of meetings with Julia, and, to me, it came to represent the arse end of the pastoral work spectrum. I didn't know anything about Derek before I saw him. I gleaned his personal details from the notes and conversations with his doctor and the nursing staff after the first encounter. It was one of those 'Can you please see if you can do anything with this patient—we've tried everything we can think of' referrals. This was just like Julia's, but that's where the resemblance ended.

Many pastoral workers who see themselves as part of a team of health professionals take reading the notes in a patient's file very seriously, as it's an important part of their practice to be as informed as possible about the patient's condition and background before they see them. And they make copious notes themselves about their interactions, in the patient's file.

I recognise this as good, sensible professional practice, in one sense—not because medical staff are that interested in what we do, but from the point of view of other pastoral workers who may be seeing that patient later, when you're off duty. But for myself, at some point in my so-called career as a pastoral worker, I decided never to read the patient's notes before seeing him or her. I wanted, rather, to learn about the person I was seeing from them, and from my own observations. I didn't want to bring all that baggage into the room with me. I wanted to be able to form my own relationship with a person, starting from scratch, and I wanted to be able to say that what was said there remained private between the two of us.

But, of course, when you're still training you can't get away with that. Every week you have to present a clinical pastoral report to the group. In it, you report significant interaction/s with a patient, and you are required to include the conversation/s you had with that patient. Each utterance is numbered and classified. You use an initial, not the person's full name in these reports; but since you're required to include details like the ward and the bed the patient is in, and the time and date of your encounter, it is hardly anonymous. Writing THIS IS A CONFIDENTIAL DOCUMENT at the top is only going to pique people's interest.

Some of the most moving and personal encounters I had were never presented in these reports, because I didn't want them to be subject to this kind of audit culture. The idea began to form in my mind that to try to make some of these encounters into rich and meaningful stories would be a way of honouring these people, so long as I respected their confidentiality by changing their names and other details. I hope I've managed to do that.

But I reported on Derek because it rocked the foundations of my newly acquired sense of competence as a certified pastoral worker, and I needed the support of my colleagues in thinking through my encounters with him:

> D. is a 40 year old man. He is not married or in a relationship and has no children. His occupation is cook.

He is said to be estranged from his family and he didn't tell anyone that he was going to hospital for a procedure but said he was going on a holiday. I knew him from a previous admission. When I visited him on [date] and introduced myself, he asked, 'What can I do for you?' in a very cold way as if I was in his shop.

[Date and time] [Ward number] [Bed number]
JK : Hello my name is Johannes. I'm the pastoral worker on this ward.
DS1 : OK. What can I do for you?
JK2 : It's more about if I can do anything for you.
DS2 : I'm fine thanks.
JK3 : OK no worries!

He was recently readmitted. He was told that no further treatment was possible and that he had between one and two months to live. He was devastated. He said he believed that he was going to be cured and that he would recover. He became very withdrawn and asked to be left alone to process the information.

I had received a referral from social work on [date], and from the patient's doctor the following day. She spoke to me at length about D. mentioning mental health issues. She said that when the ambulance went to collect him, his house was messy and dirty and he had not been caring for himself ('the house was covered in dog faeces'—doctor [date]).

On a number of occasions over the next few days I went to check on him. Mostly he was sleeping, on occasions he was with other staff, nurses, doctors, social workers, psych—never with visitors, always in bed lying flat on his back with the blankets drawn up tightly around his neck. I ensured that duty pastoral workers were aware of him in handover meetings, flagged him with the pastoral-care department representative at the pain and palliative care meeting, and on only two occasions managed to engage him in brief conversations. [dates].

When I visit Derek the second time, his eyes are closed. Did he quickly close them and pretend to be asleep when he saw me coming? I stand beside the bed for a few minutes. He opens his eyes and says angrily, 'I don't want to talk to you!'

'OK. That's OK.' But I don't move.

'I've got Nothing. To. Say to you.'

'Are you sure?'

'Yes!'

'Can I just sit with you for a while?'

'No!'

'Would you like me to come back later?'

'No.'

'Do you think you will ever want to speak to me?'

'No!' (exasperated)

'OK then, I'll leave you in peace.'

'Thank. You!'

These are the very outer limits of what you can do as a pastoral worker. You've already gone way beyond the limits that would be outlined in an imaginary pastoral-care manual. And still you feel like saying: *Come on, Derek. Talk to me! You've got two months to live … Let's talk about … something. Anything. The football. The ten-to-the-power-*

of-five-hundred universes … But … you can't. His death belongs only to him.

I only wish I knew for sure that he doesn't think I'm just a god-botherer. Sometimes I feel burdened by the title of pastoral worker. I'm convinced I'd get more traction if I was just a visitor, with no baggage and no title, who visited patients and greeted them, like when I used to sell them newspapers. But then you're not allowed to talk to them about the ten-to-the-power-of-five-hundred universes and what it means to be a human being.

Parents

'How long do you reckon I've got?' Julia asks breezily when I sit down by her bedside. I've been seeing her almost every day for six weeks.

'No idea,' I say.

She looks like she's had a reasonable night. She seems relaxed, almost playful.

'How long would you like?'

She pulls a face. 'A year?'

'You'd be happy with a year?'

She takes the plastic tube that provides the oxygen she needs out of her mouth, with her slight hand.

'*Happy*?!'

'I mean, you'd settle for that?'

She looks pensive.

'I'd like to see Daisy settle in at high school.'

We've spent hours discussing how and when to tell Daisy about her mother's illness, which now seems to have spread to her lungs.

'She starts in the new year?'

'Yes.'

'So that's in … six months, give or take—and then another six for her to settle in …'

'Yes.'

'So you'd be ha … OK … with a year?'

'Two would be better,' she says quickly, as if it's up to me.

'OK, well … you might as well aim for two years. Who knows?'

She smiles a doubtful smile. She doesn't believe it. And neither do I.

One of the things we have in common is that we are both intensely interested in how our relationships with our parents shape us. At the time I am reading Alison Bechdell's book about her mother, *Are You My Mother?* In it, she discovers the work of the psychoanalyst D.W. Winnicott, who never became as famous as Freud or Jung or Lacan, and, through her, I discover him. I develop a theory that we must all forgive our mothers, I become obsessed with it. What I learn from Winnicott, indirectly, is that you can never love your mother enough. And for my mother, nothing was ever enough.

And then I had children with another person for whom nothing was ever enough. I guess I was comfortable with people for whom nothing was ever enough, and I had myself become someone for whom nothing was ever enough, and, in that, I was like my mother. It took me a long, long time to work that one out.

Some of us hate our father and love our mother, and some of us hate our mother and love our father. Some of us begin by hating our mother and loving our father, and then we switch. At a certain age, to our great surprise, we suddenly find ourselves hating our fathers and loving our mothers—or vice versa. That's how it goes, it seems, for some of us. Then there are others who always hate both their father and their mother. And apparently there are also those who just love both their parents, or purport to do so. I guess it's possible.

I feel mostly neutral about my mother and my father now. The booze was a problem for him, and the sex. He never learned a way to contain his desire. Few people do. Mostly people just do what he did, which is whatever they can get away with. And as for my mother, as I get older, she can still make me sad, but she has less and less power to make me do what she wants. Living thirteen-and-a-half thousand kilometres away helps, with the added bonus that she doesn't like flying. So I'm safe.

Julia's mother, Ethel, lives in Western Australia—a long way away, but not far enough. Ethel arrives to visit Julia when I am with her. Julia doesn't so much ask her mother to go away because we are talking; she tells her. And Ethel does. I feel bad. I couldn't have done that to my mother. But she is different. She doesn't see Ethel's sadness. She doesn't want to see it.

'I don't like my mother.'

'Why not?'

'She was cruel!'

I want her to forgive her mother. I want her to die in peace.

A letter

I lie awake during the night thinking about how I could approach Derek.

If you don't want to talk to me, I could talk to you.

And I think of all the things I could say to him about everything that is still possible, that not all is lost. *You can still forgive your mother, Derek.*

But there is nothing I can do. I've done everything I can, by making myself available, by being present to him. When someone insists that they don't want to have anything to do with you, that's it. You have to respect that. Who would have thought this would be the hardest part of the job?

I was lucky enough to be able to leave work early that day, and I walked home. I always walk home, unless it's raining. But that day I took a route that is less than direct, and, for the first time on that grey and gloomy day, the sun came out. And I walked in the sunshine, and I looked back at the city as it receded behind me, and I felt my gratitude to be living and working here, and the sun on my back. And I felt my powerlessness, and I remembered the look of hurt in Derek's eyes. It was the look of a man who had been wronged—by the world, by life. And he was angry. And there was nothing I could do.

But Derek can still teach me something: sometimes all you can do is shed a few quiet tears for someone as you're walking home. That's all you can do, and that's not nothing, and I may well have ideas about how I could help him, but that's about me, not about him. If he is unwilling, there is nothing I can do, and I am not sure about the ethical implications of continuing to try. I have to respect his wishes and his dignity.

At three o'clock in the morning I'm lying awake thinking about Derek. Suddenly I realise I have to write him a letter. I have to write him a letter because what is keeping me awake is that I will never be able to say what I want to say to him, because he doesn't want to hear what I want to say to him. It's a letter that for professional reasons can never be sent, but I have to write it as if I *would* send it, and as if he would receive it. Lacan says the letter always arrives at its destination. The destination of this letter is myself, the aim being to get these words out of my system. It is about what I can't do, where I can't be, what I can't say.

Dear Derek

I know you don't want to talk to me and I don't expect that you will even read this but I am writing it all the same. Maybe you will wake up at three o'clock in the morning and think about me as I thought about you. And I thought about all the things I could say to you, all the things I want to say, if you'd give me a chance.

But you don't know me. You only know me as that annoying guy that keeps showing up by your bedside with a half smile who says, 'Hello, how are you going?' and then you say, 'I don't want to talk to you.' And he says, 'That's all right, that's ok.' And he says, 'I'll come back another time' and disappears quickly, before you have a chance to say 'Don't bother.'

I know about your medical situation and your prognosis. I know about your estrangement from your family. I also know about dignity and what it means. I know about a lot of other things, too, that I wish we could talk about together.

The first time I saw you, you said, 'What can I do for you?' and I thought about that for a long time. It was a stinging rebuke. It meant: state your business and then leave me alone. And when I said the word pastoral I think I saw you wince. I think if I'd said I was the child of the devil I would have got a more favourable response. For all I know you've had some terrible experiences with priests or other Christian types. For all I know you were subjected to religion by your family when you were a child, and that is why you are estranged from them.

I don't know about these things and you don't have to tell me about them. I mean, you could. I wish you would! I wish you would unburden yourself. You might find it helpful. But if you don't want to, that's ok. That's your choice. But I hope it's not because you think I'm a priest or someone who is going to try and preach to you, that you don't want to talk to me, Derek. I'm not a priest. And I'm not your father or your mother. I'm not the person who betrayed your trust.

I know you've been told the disease has progressed to the point where no further treatment, beyond trying to contain the pain, is possible. I know that this is not what you were expecting. I know that this is not what you were hoping for. I know they have given you a timeframe which is somewhat arbitrary. They are looking at the progress of the disease and how fast it has progressed in the past few months. In the light of their experience with this kind of aggressive, malignant cancer, they have given you a ball-park figure of how long you might have, and chances are that it is somewhere in that ball-park, but it could equally well be half or twice that. They just know people want to have some idea about how long they've got.

But what I want to say is that whatever the amount of time is that remains for you, it's possible to do some significant things in that time, some really meaningful, powerful, good things. In that time, Derek, you could forgive your mother. You could even apologise if you want, and you might give your mother the opportunity to apologise to you. She might want to, and you might be able to accept that apology.

I don't know the details. I don't need to know them. You don't need to tell me. You just need to know this.

Jesus died for somebody's sins

Eugene is not a nihilist. He doesn't really subscribe to any isms, other than capitalism, and probably hedonism. So that makes it doubly hard when you are no longer capable of experiencing pleasure and you're worried about what's going to happen to all that lovely money that you worked so hard to gather, when you're not there to look after it—or spend it—anymore.

And now, he doesn't know what to believe, and he's running out of time. Such is the curse of the lapsed Catholic. I don't know if there is a similar emphasis on the idea of God as a father figure in other flavours of Christianity, but for me, as a sad and lonely little Dutch boy lacking a significant patriarchal presence, it made the church quite attractive, at least for a few years. But, as a teenager, what I began to experience as the patronising paternalism of the church, increasingly repelled me.

There was something Eugene should have told his father before he died. What was it?

On a number of occasions I try to steer the conversation in the direction of the subject. I even ask him straight up one day, but he skirts around the issue, and changes the topic.

'So if your dad was still alive …' I say softly, 'and you could talk to him …' He looks at me with big eyes, as if he is channelling his inner child. '… What would you say?'

He is in the zone for a second or two before he recovers himself.

'So I suppose you just go around seeing people and you keep trying, and then sometimes you get a conversion.'

It's as if he doesn't remember when we spoke about me not being a believer, and the difference between being an atheist and an agnostic. But you never know what kind of drugs people are on in a hospital, especially if you don't read their file.

'Well … as I said before … we are all of us different, and, like I told you, I'm not a Christian.'

I try to make eye contact, but he is avoiding it.

'So I'm not looking to convert anyone. But if people are interested and they ask me what I believe, I'll tell them.'

'So what do you believe?'

I laugh. 'Boom boom … that worked!'

Eugene smiles. It worked for him, too. He successfully steered me away from the topic of what he should have told his father.

My supervisor likes to stroke his beard and say, 'Pastoral care is an art *and* a craft.' I do enjoy a pithy aphorism. When I was training as a therapist, I was told not to let people get away with the kind of move that Eugene pulled there. But the relationship between a pastoral worker and a patient in a hospital is different from that of a therapist and their client. They can get away with anything. And why shouldn't they?

In supervision, I was talking about a conversation I'd had with a patient, and my supervisor asked, 'What were you doing?'

Flustered, I responded with a flood of words about the patient and the conversation, trying to make it sound less like I was counselling them. My supervisor leaned forward, put his hand on my arm, and looked me in the eye.

'What were you *doing*?'

'I'm not sure what you mean?'

'That was Pastoral Counselling!'

Relieved, I laugh.

'Oh, OK. Is that what I was doing?'

There is an item, 'Pastoral Counselling' in the activities list when you fill in your statistics at the end of the day—or if you're me, at the end of the week—but it's rarely used, and I've never been told what it is. In fact, it was stressed in our pastoral-care training that we are *not* counsellors.

But although pastoral workers sometimes do counselling, and counsellors do sometimes do therapy—and therapists do plenty of counselling—even counselling is not therapy. I don't think of the work I do with people now, or what I did then, as therapy or counselling—it's a conversation, a particular kind of conversation that is private, one-on-one, and where I give the person all of my attention. And extraordinary things happen when you give someone all of your attention, a commodity that is becoming rarer and rarer in a world where devices and channels constantly demand it and promise instant reward when you give it. In this way it is not so different from teaching when it's done authentically, but today teaching loads are such that teachers are only rarely able (or willing) to give their full attention to one of their students.

In deciding to undergo training as a pastoral worker, I was looking for something that was *not* therapy, less hierarchical, not a case of one person having power over another, more egalitarian, and more collaborative. And that is why I resisted answering Eugene's question about what I believe.

I have no idea what people mean when they say 'spirituality', and they say it a lot in pastoral care. I have no experience of spiritual beings or a spiritual realm, except under the influence of psychedelic drugs, but that's a long time ago. I avoid the use of the word 'spiritual' except in extreme circumstances, like when I am trying to convince a review panel that I am worthy of certification as a pastoral-care practitioner, and I need a word that gestures at the topic at hand. But the idea of some kind of individual 'spiritual' essence that continues to exist after the body dies, and which remains recognisable as what that person *was*, seems a narcissistic idea. This is exactly why Heidegger argued for what he called 'being-towards-death': to be aware on a continuing basis of our mortality.

I became interested in doing this work because I wanted to look after the non-believers, the atheists, the agnostics, and the ones who *want* to believe — as in *The X Files* — but don't know in what. And what I learned as I was doing this was that non-believers have something important to learn from believers; it is not about what you believe: it's about how faith works, and how useful it is to have something to believe in, especially in a foxhole. Believing in something connects you with others, and it connects you to the past and the future.

And this is how I failed Eugene. Because that was exactly what he needed, to believe in something. And this is what a pastoral worker should be able to help with. I thought that by asking me what I believe, he was asking me what I thought *he* should believe. That's the essence of the good old, bad old-fashioned Christianity that burdened me as a youngster. They told me exactly what I ought to believe. But I didn't want to believe that, and that made me feel like a sinner. And I wanted to be good, oh Lord. I truly did. But I would regularly damn him. And allegedly every time you take the Lord's name in vain, you offend him.

I feel like that about the word 'love' now. I rarely use it, because it suffers from overuse. And nine hundred and ninety-nine times out of a thousand, it is taken in vain.

It was not until Patti Smith told me that Jesus didn't, in fact, die for my sins, but somebody else's and released me … redeemed me … with her shambolic shaman act and goddamn, *goddamn,* here I am, too … that I realised I was a lost sheep on a vast continent of disbelief.

The hand of God

I receive a referral for Natalie the day after I give up on Derek.

'She has cancer of the vulva, and she's been crying all night,' the nurse says *sotto voce*. We've paused just outside one of the ward's single rooms. 'She's in a lot of pain. We're trying to make her comfortable, but ...' She makes a face. 'Poor dear. She's 87!'

You can get cancer in your vulva?!

I barely have time to digest the idea before I'm in a room that reeks of urine, with a tiny figure, partially covered by a blanket, sitting next to the bed weeping. The nurse introduces me. Natalie barely looks up. She is holding a rosary in one hand, and I take the other hand in mine.

'Is that the hand of God ... or is that your hand?' she whispers.

I think for a moment.

'It's my hand.'

Natalie looks at me for the first time. Her eyes are blue.

'Will I go tonight?'

It takes me several seconds to process what she is asking me. The eyes are looking at me expectantly.

'It's possible. Yes. Or tomorrow night. Or when you're ready. Are you ready?'

'Yes.'

'Is there anything you need to say to anyone?'

'No.'

She weeps soundlessly.

Of all the ten-to-the-power-of-five-hundred universes I could be in, I am in this one.

'Did God send you to me?' Natalie whispers.

There is only one possible answer.

'Yes.'

There is no room for an atheist in this foxhole.

Reality therapy

Every day as a pastoral worker brings its own unique challenges. Working out what is required of you each day furthers progress with your work on the project of being human, according to Hannah Arendt, or living an authentic life, as her teacher Martin Heidegger had it—and the project is never finished. The project truly is, and will remain, what as artists we liked to call 'work in progress' (regardless of whether it actually is).

As a pastoral worker, your job is to engage people in conversation. That's number one. The difference between talking and not talking is huge. The actual topic of the conversation doesn't matter so much. It is having someone to talk to in the hospital that can make such a difference to someone's experience of illness. Sometimes a cancer diagnosis will lead a person to consider what is important in life, and what it means to be a human being, and to begin to articulate that problem. Someone might experience an urgent conscious or unconscious need to tell someone who they are and what it means to be them.

I learned this in Germany, in a place the Germans call a *kurort*—literally, a place to get cured—at Bad Bentheim, just across the Dutch–German border. I had just completed an intensive training course in reality therapy. As a former postmodernist cynic and battle-hardened academic, I had found the idea of reinventing myself as a reality therapist mildly amusing and kind of apt. What I didn't realise was that I would learn how to listen, how to *be* a listener.

I never had trouble talking to people—or I thought I didn't—but I wanted to talk with them about things that are important. I'm not someone who enjoys talking about myself, and I found it excruciating to have to listen to people talking about *themselves*. I didn't find the minutiae of people's lives interesting, and I was always waiting for them to get to the point. But what I didn't realise was that people *need* to talk about themselves in order to feel like they exist. I became aware that often, when people were talking to me, I was nodding and smiling—or scowling, as the case may be, if they were being boring—but my brain was busy thinking about something else, and I was not giving them my full attention.

Immediately following the reality-therapy course, I got on a plane to Germany to be with my mother, who was entering a German hospital to have a new knee fitted, followed by a month of rehabilitation in Bad Bentheim, and it became my own kind of *kurort*.

During my six weeks in Germany I began practising how to engage people in conversations and listening. I also had to practise being an optimist for my mother's sake. For the first time in my life, I had the upper hand in my relationship with her. And for the first time, I was of use to her, but on my own terms, not hers. And I think it was on one of those cold, dark nights, as I cycled back to the hotel from the hospital on my borrowed bicycle through the snow and the rain with Bruce Springsteen in my headphones, that I finally forgave my mother.

Pauli's exclusion principle

Every person I saw in the hospital during my year of training who was able to talk about what was important to them was in better spirits than those who could not or would not talk. But then the nihilists wouldn't talk to me in any case because I was a pastoral worker, and a pastoral worker is like a walking advertisement for faith — even if their faith, like mine, consists of something much more nebulous than a belief in a supernatural being or an afterlife. An angry man called Lionel said to me, 'About the last thing I feel like doing is talking to a pastoral worker about the you-knee-verse.' He pronounced 'the universe' in an exaggerated way, like Brian Cox, but he said it like he had nothing but contempt for it.

I was not fan of D:Ream, the eighties pop band that Brian Cox was a member of, but after the band broke up he morphed into a professor of physics, and is now frequently seen on BBC-TV programs enthusing about some aspect of the universe, and he is the author of books with titles like *Everything That Can Happen Does Happen*.

Brian is cute, but he has an annoying way of pronouncing the word 'universe'. He says it like this: 'you-knee-verse,' emphasising each of the three syllables. And he says it a lot. But there is something compelling in Brian's explanations of quantum physics, and one day I find that I am somehow consoled by Pauli's exclusion principle, according to which—or, at least, this is the way Brian explains it—every single subatomic particle in the entire universe is connected to every other subatomic particle, since no particle can have exactly the same quantum state (energy level, position, and momentum) as any other particle. Thus if an atom changes its energy state (and this is not an infrequent event), its constituent elements have to be 'aware' of the quantum state of the constituent elements of every other atom in the entire universe.

So each atom in my body is connected to each and every other atom in the universe.

To me, this means that when the person formerly known to me as 'I' is dead, every single one of the electrons which formerly constituted that 'I' will continue to be connected to every other electron in the universe. And now and here, that 'I' is connected to every other human and non-human being, and every living and non-living 'thing'. Sometimes when I'm very quiet, I imagine that I'm conscious or aware, to some very minimal but not insignificant extent, of that connection.

But Brian doesn't like people drawing their own conclusions about the implications of quantum physics and what it might mean for their understanding and experience of reality. To be sure, there are all kinds of oddballs out there who will utilise some aspect of quantum theory for their own purposes, but Brian should read Roland Barthes. Just as someone somewhere is sampling D:Ream, some of us take comfort in the idea that everything is connected, and that we exist in one (or several) of ten-to-the-power-of-five-hundred universes—or a quantum universe—where everything is possible, and where everything that can happen does happen. Brian is right, and he himself is evidence of it.

So I was unusual for a pastoral worker, not only for being, I suppose, an atheist—although I'd rather think of myself as a non-believer—but because I believe in a kind of immortality. Perhaps 'belief' is too strong a word, and so is 'immortality.' It's not as though I believe that 'I' stay intact or survive somehow after my death, although with any luck some of these words might persist for a while. We are, after all, constituted by language.

When I told Julia about Pauli and the eleven dimensions and the ten-to-the-power-of-five-hundred universes, she looked incredulous.

'But there are only a few scientists who believe that.'

That's true, but to me it is a more intriguing idea than the idea of an authoritarian, omnipresent being. Still, I'm not evangelistic. I have no doubt that we are all connected in some ineffable way to each other, to all the other living and non-living things, and to the entirety of what is in each of the ten-to-the-power-of-five-hundred universes and the eleven dimensions, but I keep quiet about it.

In any case, I don't know what else to say about it because it is elusive, and everything you say about something that is ineffable is too much. And, if you ask me what I believe in, I would rather talk in terms of ethics and the need to address the problem of poverty and inequality in the world, and the suffering and misery of so many beings. If you want to call that a 'faith', so be it. It has a similar effect. I know what it's like to be consoled by what you believe.

The second coming

Giovanni has the kind of eyebrows seen almost exclusively on elderly gentlemen from southern Europe — furrowed, with a lot of hairs in many and various shades ranging from black to grey, growing in different directions, a number of them quite recalcitrant. He wants me to go to the TAB to put some money on 'the gee-gees' for him, and I say no. Giovanni is the kind of elderly southern European gentleman who is used to having things his own way. He winked and smiled when he was asking me, but as soon as I said no, his face clouded over and he avoided eye contact. Yesterday he was keen for a newspaper, and now I know why. He'd missed the shop trolley because they were having trouble with his catheter and he was off the ward having it fixed. It was late in the day, and he looked bored and annoyed. He speaks virtually no English, or it suits him to make you think so.

I don't like the *Herald Sun*, but when I sold newspapers on the wards in another hospital (that seems like a lifetime ago, and I guess it was), I sold ten copies of the *Herald Sun* for every copy of the *Age*, and sometimes more. By the end of my shift I'd always run out of the *Herald Sun*, and I'd say, 'I've got the *Age* ...' and they'd scowl. The average *Herald Sun* reader would rather not have a newspaper at all than read the *Age*. I suspect an *Age* reader would make do with a

Herald Sun if push came to shove, but how would you know?

'Which paper do you want, Giovanni?' I ask.

'*Herald Sun.*'

'What if I can only get the *Age*? Do you want the *Age*?'

'*Herald Sun*,' he says angrily.

'Yeah, but what if they've sold out? I might only be able to get the *Age* at this time of day.'

'*Herald Sun!*'

He waves me away. He doesn't want to think about the possibility that the *Herald Sun* may have sold out.

During my time in the foxhole I talk to people with a wide range of beliefs, prejudices, and ideologies, as well as to people who refuse to believe things, such as that their cancer is terminal. It's quite possible to die whilst refusing to believe that you're dying. I'd always thought there would come a point where you'd have to accept the inevitable, but it seems that you don't. The inevitable will happen anyway. Some believe in their own luck or willpower. Others believe that making their body alkaline will cure their cancer, and they employ some peculiar eating habits to try to make it so.

Within seconds of introducing myself to yet another angry-looking southern European gentleman on the ward, he is telling me about the second coming.

'It will take place in the next five to ten years.'

I've been warned about him at handover. 'He'll talk your head off about the second coming ...', one of my colleagues, who is a committed Christian, said, rolling her eyes and making a face. I would have liked to ask why the second coming was any more unbelievable to her than some of the things she does believe in, but handover was not the time.

Maybe there is no good time to ask someone why they believe one thing rather than another, or refuse to believe one thing and not another. Perhaps some of us are just more disposed to believing, or refusing to believe, than others.

He is just about to tell me more when the phone rings. He apologises.

'I have to take this call.'

'That's OK,' I say, quite relieved.

'You can tell me more next time!'

But there isn't to be a next time. He is discharged before I can see him again. So I'm afraid I haven't any more specific details about the second coming. As far as I know, it hasn't happened yet. But how would you know? It won't be in the *Age* or the *Herald Sun*.

The newspaper shelf in the shop is bare. There isn't even an *Age* to be had. I walk around the hospital looking for a discarded newspaper for Giovanni in the deserted waiting rooms in Radiotherapy and in the Chemical Day Unit. I even check the bins. Nothing. When I go back to give Giovanni the bad news, he is asleep.

Now that I have reached an age which people under thirty think is old, I feel increasingly like I am surrounded by ever-growing numbers of nihilists, and not just any old nihilists, not the good old devil-may-care, good-humoured kind, but passive-aggressive nihilists who hate anyone who believes in anything, and anyone who has any hope for the future or the possibility of a better world. That's not just zero — that is zero to the power of zero.

And when they land in the hospital, there is nothing that can be done with them because they refuse to engage. They refuse to have their wounds dressed. They refuse to have their stoma changed. They refuse to have a shower or be washed. They are, without a doubt, the least popular people in the hospital. That was Derek to a tee. And that is why Christians are afraid of atheists: they think all atheists are nihilists, and there are plenty that are. They are also cynics and pessimists—a dangerous combination.

What I should have told Eugene

And then I realise what I should have told Eugene. I should have told him that what I believe in is living an ethical life, an authentic life, and that philosophy and quantum theory are my consolations. And this is why I sometimes say I'm an agnostic—not about an omnipotent supernatural being, but about the possibility that the connection between the electrons that constitute me and every other electron in the ten-to-the-power-of-five-hundred universes is meaningful in some way that my mind is too small to contain, or because my brain is not doing one-hundred-thousandth of what it is capable of, or probably would have been capable of, if a previous version of me had not destroyed all those brain cells with alcohol and drugs.

And what I should have told him is that all of this leads me to believe that whilst I am a being-towards-death, there is something beyond the cold, empty, rational world, beyond the world of common sense, that we don't have any inkling of, because our current ways of thinking about reality are not able to accommodate it. Somewhere in the eleven dimensions and the ten-to-the-power-of-five-hundred universes there is something *huge*, something ineffable, mysterious, magical. But I'm an existential detective, and not a magician, although I do believe that everything is possible.

And what I should have told him was, I believe that in one hundred years, or two or three hundred years from now, people will look back at this time and the way we live and think now, and the way we conduct our lives and the way we allow people to suffer at the end of their lives, and they will sadly shake their heads, and sigh and say: 'If only they had known.'

And what I should have told Eugene was that I believe we are on the verge of discovering a radically different way of understanding and thinking about reality and the world and the universe, and what it means to be a human being. I don't mean this is going to happen next week. It is going to take generations — probably centuries, maybe even a thousand years — for us to fully comprehend and act on and discover the implications of what quantum physics began to uncover one hundred years ago. There are a few of us who have an inkling of this. I am not one of them, but I have read some books by people who do have an inkling, and some of what they are saying I can begin to understand, and I believe them.

Maybe what I should have told Eugene was that there is a mystery which we cannot understand, which we cannot fathom, cannot apprehend, but there is a place you can go using your mind where you can allow for that possibility, and what it means to go there is that you don't have to die in a cold, rational, meaningless universe. And whilst you and

I will both die like primitive beings without the capacity to understand the nature of *what is*, it will nevertheless alter your relationship with the world and everything in it, and you will be peaceful. But maybe I was worried that in the end he would be sorry he had asked. Maybe he was looking for someone just to say, 'I believe God will forgive you,' and I was not the right person for that job.

Eulogy

The good-enough mother

I arrive at the hospital to find that Julia has been moved to the intensive-care unit overnight. This means that her condition has worsened significantly. On the ward, the expectation is that we are going to lose her. As I make my way down to intensive care, I realise for the first time what her dying will mean to me. But when I get to the ICU, Julia is sitting in a chair, wearing her pink hat, and she greets me with a half-smile and a question.

'So, if you were dying, what would be the top five things that you'd want to do before you die?'

There are no other patients in the ICU.

'Hmm, that's a good question.' I swallow hard. There is a lump in my throat that won't go down.

'You mean, after I'd said the things that I want to say to the people I love and care about?'

'Yes.'

'And have you done that?'

'Yes.' There is sadness in that smile.

'And are you continuing to do that?

'Yes.'

'Because that's an ongoing thing, isn't it, that you need to continue doing?'

There is a pause.

'Yes.'

'Well, then, I've always had the idea that I wanted to write a book. So depending on how much time I had left, I would want to try and do that.'

'I often have ideas for a book,' Julia says brightly. 'Do you think I have a book in me?'

'Well, they say everyone has one book in them. What would your book be about?'

'Just about my life, I guess, my memories—a memoir.'

'OK.'

'It all sounds great echoing around in my head, but writing it down would be more difficult.'

'Why is that?'

'Because then it would be under scrutiny, open to criticism.'

'Whose criticism would you be particularly worried about?'

'My mother.'

'Is she very critical of you in general?'

'Yes. She's gone back to Perth now, thank God. But I gave her a piece of my mind before she went.'

'Really? What were you giving her a piece of your mind about?'

'Her partner. He is the controlling type. They were going away for the weekend, and then he changed his mind and she was whinging. And I said, "Just go by yourself then." And she said, "Oh no, George wouldn't like that." And I told her off. Tom would have come with me if I wanted to go!'

'Do you think our parents ever take any notice of advice we give them?'

'Probably not.'

'Would forgiving your mother be one of the things on your list?'

'No. She was too cruel.'

'My mother said an awful thing to me once. She didn't so much say it, as scream it at me, from another room. I don't know if it would have been better or worse if I'd been in the same room. If I had been, she probably wouldn't have been able to get the words out.'

'What did she say?'

'It's too awful. I can't bring myself to repeat it. Think of the worst thing your mother could say to you, and multiply it by a hundred.'

'But you have forgiven her?'

'Yeah.'

'That's amazing.'

'Well, I don't know. I had no choice.'

'You have a choice!'

'I think you can believe you've got a choice, but you don't have a choice. You *have to* forgive your mother.'

'You think?'

'Without a doubt!'

We are silent now. She looks tired, and sad.

'Let's leave it here today.' I say. 'You want to rest?'

'OK.'

'I'll come and see you tomorrow?'

She takes my proffered hand, and holds it.

'Yes, please.' She smiles wearily.

'OK!'

I think there are many people in the world who are cruel to others because they are unable to forgive their mothers (or fathers) for being cruel to *them*, and they are unable to access their compassion. And everyone has something to forgive their mother for. I am interested in Jung's idea of individuation, particularly the way he identifies the importance of the individual's fully realised separation from the mother and father. And I speculate that in order to fully individuate and become complete subjects in our own right and to become authentic beings, we have to forgive our mothers. And possibly our fathers. I wouldn't know about that. My father needed to be forgiven for being absent, but that's not hard. Absence is not cruelty. You can only be cruel if you are there.

D.W. Winnicott's idea of the 'good-enough mother' seems especially pertinent in a culture where motherhood is often idealised to the point of absurdity. What is a perfect mother? Who can say that their mother was perfect? In order to be able to develop a healthy sense of self, Winnicott says, what we need is not a perfect mother, but a *good-enough* mother.

It took me a long time to be able forgive my mother. I was in my late forties by then. But it was when I realised that I needed to do it, that I had no choice, that I found myself able to do it, that I was free. And so, in a way, was she—although I am not sure she experiences it that way.

No way to live

Julia tells me that the latest X-rays show shadows on her lungs. It could be pneumonia, but there aren't any other symptoms of that, like fever. Breathing is increasingly difficult for her, and she doesn't even have the energy to go to the toilet by herself.

'This is no way to live …' she sighs.

'No.'

She says she would prefer to end her life rather than live like this.

'But I'm not there yet,' she says.

'Are you afraid?'

'No … Not anymore.'

We talk about fear and about how it dissipates.

'I am just tired, that's all.'

'Yes. Fear takes energy.'

Suddenly, she looks at me intently.

'Have you ever been diagnosed with a life-threatening illness?'

'I was diagnosed with lupus once. Wrongly, as it turned out.'

I remember more about the reactions of the people I told, the ones who knew what lupus was, rather than my own, which was just numbness. I was stunned, really. But there was no fear or anger.

'I was afraid when I was first diagnosed.' Julia says. 'And then I was angry.'

'And now?'

'And now? I'm sad!' she says angrily, and weeps.

'What is your sadness about?'

'I feel like I've failed them, like I am letting them down. Daisy … and Tom …'

'No, no, no …' I put my hand on her thin arm. 'It's not

your fault that you've got this disease. You didn't choose it!'

When I reach for the box of tissues on her bedside table, the pink button I gave her a few days ago is still there.

When I'd handed it to her, what I'd said was: 'This looks like an ordinary button, but it isn't.'

Julia had taken the button from me and held it in her hand, but without giving me her full attention. I'd felt foolish, but as I'd started I had to keep going.

'This button is to remind you of a certain conversation we had. When you see it, you will be reminded of it.'

Today, instead of the tissue box, I take the button from the bedside table and hand it to her.

'It's working.' She smiles through her tears.

We talk about what it is to be an ethical person, what that means. We talk about her daughter, and what it is like to have to think about the possibility of not being there for her. She weeps.

'I think nine-tenths of the work I have to do with her is done ...'

'With Daisy?'

She nods.

I want to ask her about the part that remains undone, but I have to go to a staff meeting.

'I am off duty now until Monday, but I'll come back and see you then, OK?'

'I'd like that.'

'OK.'

'See you. Take care.'

She looks up at me. It's as if she hasn't finished with me. Always in a hospital, when we are standing up, a person who is in a bed is looking up at us. And we are looking down on them. I sit down again.

'You're the one that makes me cry,' she says softly, half to herself, 'but then I feel better.'

Discharge

So this is how it happens.

Julia is suddenly discharged one morning. It is pure coincidence—or, if you were a Jungian, you'd say it was synchronicity—that I even get to say goodbye. I am late for work. I am never late for work. If you believed in such things, you'd say it was meant to be. If I hadn't happened to be walking past on this morning, she would not have been there when I went to the ward, and I would not have seen her again. Or not until the next time she was admitted, if there is a next time.

Instead, I come across a man loading a wheelchair into the back of a car. *Hang on! That's Tom. And that's Julia in the passenger seat!* She gets out of the car.

'I'm so glad I got to see you,' she says. 'I was going to ring you.'

We hug awkwardly. It's one of those cold, sunless Melbourne winter days. In Europe, people get depressed because this kind of weather goes on for months and months. Here we shrug. She asks if I do home visits. My answer should be, *No, sorry, we can't do that.*

We're here to provide pastoral care to hospital patients,

and thus our relationships with people end when their stay in hospital ends. We don't have the resources to provide pastoral care after discharge, even though it is often much needed.

What I say is, 'Yes, of course. And, anyway, I want to see that funky place of yours!' She is not dressed for spending any amount of time outside, and I am worried about her catching a cold.

'I can get your details from the system!'

But she insists on writing her name and address and three telephone numbers in tiny longhand on a small piece of paper on the bonnet of the car. I watch the letters being laboriously formed—the ink will not flow freely. She mutters 'Fuck' under her breath.

'There. It's done.' She hands it to me.

I still have the piece of paper. I remember the skin on her thin arm reacting to the cold as she was writing. Even a dying person has a definite sense of where they live. I had never known her in her home. To me, she was a person who lived in the hospital, at my place of work. It is as if, in writing down where she lived, she was claiming her independent personhood. It is as if she was saying, 'I am still here.'

Kylie

'If you wouldn't mind seeing Kylie in 9C,' Eve says when I get to the ward. I follow her as she steps into the entrance of the handover room and lowers her voice whilst continuing to speak quickly and in dot points.

'So, she's 40, in a stable relationship with several children, recent diagnosis. She's teary, not coping at all well with being in the hospital.'

'Sure. Thanks, Eve.'

Kylie is sitting in a chair by her bed, wearing Mr. Men pyjamas, looking out of the window. They are all there: Mr. Noisy, Mr. Tickle, Mr. Bounce, and my favourite, Mr. Grumpy. After some preliminary niceties about the weather and how it can make a difference to your mood if you wear cheerful pyjamas, Kylie tells me she's upset about her sister-in-law, who was recently diagnosed with a brain tumour and is due to have surgery next week.

It's not her own diagnosis she is worried about.

'And how is she?'

'That's the thing. I don't know,' Kylie sighs. 'We had a falling out nineteen years ago, and we've never spoken since.'

'Wow—nineteen years!'

'Yeah …'

'And so are you still angry with her about what happened nineteen years ago?'

'Um … Not sure. It's a long time ago. But it's awkward. And now I'm in here, and there is nothing I can do.'

She is weeping quietly. A well-used tissue appears, and she dabs at her eyes.

'There *is* something you can do!' She looks at me.

'Why don't you ring her?'

It seems almost too obvious, and I'm expecting her to say: 'Oh, no, I couldn't do that,' and then to have a discussion with her, teasing out why not. To my complete surprise, she says, 'OK … um … I suppose I could.'

She is examining her tissue.

'But I wouldn't know what to say.'

'Well, you could say, "Look—what happened nineteen years ago happened, but right now I want to say I am thinking of you, and I hope everything goes well with your operation." And then, if she doesn't want to talk to you, that's fine. Then you could say, "I just wanted to ring and tell you that."'

She weeps. We sit together in silence for a few minutes, and then she looks at me.

'That's a really good idea. I'll do that tonight.'

'How did you go?' I ask Kylie when I'm doing my ward round the next day. She is sitting up in bed, looking chirpy. Her pyjamas have hundreds of yellow, smiley faces today.

'I was hoping you'd come by!'

She looks like a different person.

'I rang her, and it was good! She said, "I want to apologise for what happened."'

'Fantastic! And did you say, "I forgive you"?'

'Yes, I did. And she said: "Thank you." She was so happy that I rang.'

She is beaming.

'I want to thank you for your suggestion.' She takes my hand. 'A huge weight has been lifted off my shoulders.'

I am relieved. But I know full well I didn't follow protocol. That was risky, and it could have been disastrous. It could have been very upsetting for Kylie. An experienced worker would have taken a more hands-off approach, enabling Kylie to think of ringing her sister-in-law herself. I was just lucky that it turned out well. The real aim of my suggestion was to get Kylie to articulate the problem more clearly, not to solve it for her. But then, when she said, 'I suppose I could,' I guess I got carried away.

I miss Julia. Since working with her, I've thought a great deal about the importance of forgiveness, especially when you know you're going to die, or when someone who has wronged you is going to die. It's a great gift to forgive someone who has wronged you and who is remorseful before they die — or before you die. But such an act of generosity is only meaningful whilst you're both still alive, because forgiveness is a loop. You can only forgive someone who would like to be forgiven and who is remorseful about the wrong he or she did. Someone has to be prepared to receive the gift of forgiveness.

Still … forgiveness is a big word. If I was about to undergo a potentially life-ending surgical procedure, and someone I'd wronged in the past rang me to say they were thinking of me and that they were prepared to let bygones be bygones, I'd be delighted. That would be enough. But putting yourself in someone else's position is not textbook pastoral care, or textbook therapy.

When you've been diagnosed with cancer, and you're in a state of uncertainty about the future and feeling utterly disempowered, with no control over your destiny, it can affect your ability to think and to make decisions. What we should be aiming for is to help people feel empowered. We are not here to solve their problems. I'll have to be more careful about that.

The Bridge

I don't know what I was expecting from the documentary about people who kill themselves by jumping off the Golden Gate Bridge in San Francisco that I was watching on TV tonight, but it wasn't appropriate viewing for someone trying to relax after a big day at the hospital.

Everything in the universe is falling. Brian Cox told me this. But I don't want to know about the universe today.

It's not the best way to end your life, but it sure makes for a grand gesture. There are those who crawl into a corner and die quietly by themselves, and then there are those who want to make a big statement, like my friend Marcel, who set himself on fire. It is because of him and what he did that I am doing this. And I do want to see the other half of *The Bridge*—but not today.

Why was today so exhausting? I was on day duty, and there was an emergency on my ward first thing in the morning before I'd even taken off my coat and put my bag down, and then there were medical emergencies galore all day.

It's such a flawed film, so disappointing in so many ways. But it's impossible not to be interested in it because of the compassion you have for the people who jump, and the ones who are standing there and look like they're thinking about jumping. Why do they choose to do it in *this* way?

Oh, and I guess that I just don't know.

D.W. Winnicott says, 'Acceptance of not-knowing produces tremendous relief.' Ideally this would be something you learn in childhood, but it took me a long time. It was part of my mid-life crisis. Although I'm not sure I would call it a crisis—it was more like a catharsis.

I guess a non-atheist gets to acceptance of not-knowing by trusting in God, but for the rest of us it's more complicated. It is a case of believing that we know what we need to know, and that what we don't know is unlikely to hurt us.

In the hospital, there are those who want to know everything there is to know about their disease and their treatment. They say to the nurse who is about to give them an injection, 'Why are you giving me another dose of that drug? I'm on ten units a day!'

And there are those who want to know nothing.

Acceptance of not-knowing is also connected to humility, and I never had much of that before my mid-life catharsis, either. My devoutly Christian supervisor asks what I mean by humility.

'Does it mean letting people walk all over you?' she asks.

This is one of those metaphors.

'Do you mean letting people humiliate you?' she continues.

How do you stop someone humiliating you? You can make yourself feel better about it by saying to them, 'Don't humiliate me'. But is saying that not a bit humiliating in itself?

'What is the *opposite* of humility?' I ask.

'Is it confidence?'

Sometimes these supervision sessions are like two people thinking out loud together.

'I wonder if … the opposite of humility is arrogance…?' I say.

So maybe what I mean by humility is modesty, being unassuming, but not without confidence.

I spend about half an hour with Kevin and his wife, on

my ward, and about an hour with young Craig, in the next room. Craig is ten years younger than me. His prognosis is not good, but he doesn't know it yet. Or maybe he does. I run into his dad, Ian, in the corridor, and I say, 'He's a trooper, your boy. Where does his get his strength from?'

'From his grandfather!' Ian says with a big, booming voice, as if he's calling out to his cattle from across the paddock.

Keith

Today I am seeing Keith, 51, who is a new admission on my ward. He was seen by the duty pastoral worker last night in response to a referral from the nurse in charge. She flagged him as having a 'transient lifestyle'. I have no idea what this means. It could mean 'drifter', or someone who lives in a caravan park. It could refer to any of a range of non-standard and/or non-conformist attitudes to life and living. But I suspect that here it means someone who has abused alcohol and tobacco, or other 'substances'.

I feel some trepidation. I've not had much success with men who fit that description. They are generally in the hospital for cancer in a part of the body that is related to their excesses, and sometimes they are suffering from withdrawal. They can be grumpy and rough as guts, and they are not generally interested in talking about the you-knee-verse with a pastoral worker.

A clean, good-looking man, fully dressed in nice clothes, is sitting on a chair by the empty bed when I enter the room.

Keith's brother, perhaps, or another family member?

'Hello. I'm looking for Keith, but I see he's not there,' I say to the man, pointing at the empty bed.

'Yes he is!' He looks at me with a smile.

'Oh! Are … you Keith?'

'I am!'

I introduce myself. He looks so unlike any of the 'transient lifestyle' men I've met in the hospital before that I am a little taken aback.

'How did you get my name?' Keith asks.

This is an odd question.

'I work here. I have a ward list!' I hold up my list. 'But my colleague who talked with you last night …?'

He looks confused.

'She checked in with you when you were admitted?'

He obviously doesn't remember.

'Anyway, I'm the pastoral worker on this ward, and I just wanted to see how you are going …'

He nods vaguely.

'So … how *are* you going?'

'Yeah, I am going OK … I guess … I'm just … waiting for my sister. She's taking me out to lunch.'

'Oh, nice! It's a good day for it. Or … well, at least it has stopped raining,' I say brightly.

'Yes.'

'Where are you going for lunch?

'An Italian place. They do really good pasta.'

There is something enigmatic about him, with his clean-shaven face — it takes work, a shave like that. There is a kind of bemused sadness, and his eyes sparkle with intelligence. He is fiddling with something, a hat. He is looking for something.

'What are you looking for?'

'My iPad ... Oh, there it is.'

He puts it in his bag. It's a special iPad satchel. He clears some things off the chair next to him, and invites me to sit down.

'So, can you tell me what is happening for you?'

'Well, the disease has spread from my lungs to my brain. They're going to operate and take out the tumour.'

He points at his head, which is completely bald. But it is not a default baldness. It is a man making a statement, using the shape of his skull.

'And how does that make you feel?'

Suddenly he explodes with anger.

'That is such a stupid question!'

He scoffs. He repeats my words scornfully,

'"How does that make you feel?"! Do they teach you that at social-work school?' He looks at me angrily.

I am quite calm. I go into damage-control mode.

'I'm sorry. It wasn't my intention to upset you. The reason I asked you that is because some people find it helpful to talk about how they feel about their disease.'

'Well, I don't like talking about my feelings.'

'No worries at all. We don't have to talk about that.'

His anger seems to subside quite quickly. He says something I don't quite catch about his 'former life.'

'What sort of things do you like to do?'

He says nothing.

'TV? Reading?'

'My brain tumour makes it difficult for me to read.'

We sit in silence for some time.

'Do you mind if I sit here with you for a while?'

'No, that's OK … I suppose …'

He is very fidgety.

'Is it making you uncomfortable me sitting here? I can go if you don't want me here.'

'It's OK.' He points at his head. 'It's difficult for me to communicate with people because of the tumour.'

'I'm happy to keep you company while you are waiting for your sister,' I say meekly, 'but if you'd rather be alone, I can leave you in peace …'

He just says nothing. It is as if he hasn't heard me. I am looking for a way back in. I'm trying to think of a way to repair the damage, but I am not sure that I can. I should just leave him alone. But I feel like he needs something, and I am unable to give it, or even work out what it is. Eventually, I manage to get out of him that my sitting there is making him uncomfortable. So I thank him for his time, and wish him all the best.

But maybe I was the one who was uncomfortable. He was right. It was a stupid question. I was being lazy when I used the 'How does that make you feel' question. If I had been fully present, I wouldn't have asked it. It would have been obvious. Being present is everything. Each person is unique. There are general principles in working with human beings, but there is no technique or method. You have to let go of all your preconceived ideas and notions for each new encounter with every person in the hospital.

I go back to the office for a cup of tea and to lick my wounds. I console myself by remembering that I'd remained calm. I'd explained to him why I'd asked the question, and I'd apologised for upsetting him. I'd behaved professionally. I'd been competent. Yet I'd failed. I was not able to be of use.

The following Monday, I pay Keith another visit. 'I heard you're going in to have your brain surgery tomorrow.'

'It's today!'

'OK, well, I won't ask how it makes you feel!'

He says nothing. It's hard to tell from his inscrutable, immaculate face if he even remembers our conversation.

'I've been thinking about you, and I thought, "I'd like to have a conversation with you."'

'Well, I'm not much of a conversationalist, I'm afraid.'

Again, that expressionless face. I wish him well, and he smiles. He is relieved, probably, that I'm finally going to leave him alone. He thanks me for visiting him.

On the way back to the office, I meet Julia and Tom in the street. She is arriving for an MRI scan, and is feeling good. The conversation turns to Daisy. They want her to have a meeting with the counsellor, but Daisy doesn't want to go.

'Is this a pastoral issue or a counselling issue?' Julia asks.

The street is not an ideal place for a meta discussion on the difference between therapy and pastoral care, especially with this cold wind blowing and big clouds packing in. The work I'd want do with Daisy would be aimed at forgiving Julia whilst she is still alive. But that's not likely to be possible in the time she has left, even if they were to trust me enough to let me work with their daughter. That work will have to come later, many years from now—maybe when she is as old as her mother is now. And she'll probably have to pay a lot of money to a psychoanalyst to get to it.

We arrange for me to do the house call on Sunday, and I've been promised cakes from Julia's favourite French patisserie. I could have asked for special permission to see her at home—but I didn't. The powers that be might have said no, and there is urgent, unfinished business. I still need to help her work out how to tell her daughter what is by now abundantly, overwhelmingly clear. It's not a question of 'your mother is going to die,' but 'your mother is dying.' How do you help a mother tell her child that she is going to die, and that it will be sooner rather than later—and how do you tell a child that she has to forgive her mother for dying?

Vilma

Vilma is reading a magazine when I pause by her bed to say hello. She looks up from her reading and, with a sad smile asks, or rather *urges,* me to sit down.

'Sit down! Sit down!'

She carefully folds her magazine and puts it in the drawer. She was diagnosed six years ago, she tells me, so she feels she's done pretty well, and says how proud she is of her two sons and two grandsons. Vilma brought up the two kids alone.

No doubt there is a tragic story there, but today it's a different tragedy that Vilma wants to relate. It's the one about her brother, Fransz. He came out to Australia with her in 1958. The year of my birth.

I smile. 'A very good year!'

She smiles.

'A very clever boy with an engineering degree from back home ...'

Her voice is slightly clipped, but the intonations are more melodic than a German accent would be.

'... from Czechoslovakia ...'

She is silent for a few moments.

'A year after we got here, he was in a car accident. Completely paralysed.'

She looks at me intently to see if those two words have had an impact, and they do. Hearing some people's life stories makes you feel like you're staring into an abyss.

So she looked after her brother, as well as her two boys, and then it was just her and Fransz at home. The children were grown up and married, with good jobs and children of their own. What worried her, when she was diagnosed, was not herself or the children, but who was going to look after Fransz. And then Fransz, too, was diagnosed with cancer, and there was nothing they could do for him, it was so far advanced. So they just made him comfortable, she says, and then he got pneumonia and died.

'On the last day, he kept looking out of the window as if he was waiting for something or someone,' she tells me sadly. 'I said, "Fransz ... Fransz, what are you looking at?" But by this time he could no longer speak.'

When they went to pick up the ashes from Springvale, they couldn't find them.

'They were looking for them everywhere ...' she almost whispers, and moves in a little closer, as if she is about to tell me a secret. 'And you know where we found them?'

Of course she knows that I don't know, but she looks at me with a feigned expectancy, as if we're actors in a play.

'You tell me what this means ...' she says, and pauses a moment for effect. 'We found them at the number of the house where we were born!'

I am confused.

'You tell me what it means,' she demands with a half-smile.

'What does it mean to you?' I ask, smiling back.

'He was giving me a message!'

She folds and refolds the handkerchief that she took out of the drawer when she began telling me about Fransz, perhaps in anticipation of tears, but none came.

'He was telling me he wanted to go home.'

I am incredulous, but I am nodding.

'So we sent his ashes back to Slovakia, and we had a cousin scatter them,' she says wistfully. 'I still dream about him. A few weeks ago, I dreamed about him, and I said, "Fransz, how are you ... Are you all right?" and he looked wonderful! Just like he used to ... before the accident. And he said, "I am at peace."'

'Wow.'

'Yes. That is what he told me ... in the dream, you know. You tell me what it means,' she says again.

I smile. 'Next time,' I say, 'I will tell you about the message my grandmother sent me when she died.'

'What was it?'

'I'll have to tell you next time. I have to go now.'

She looks disappointed, but says, 'OK' and goes back to her magazine.

I should have stayed and told her. The next day, she was discharged. I hoped to see Vilma's tragic smile and her determined face again. You never know in here. But you also kind of hope you don't see people again. It's not usually good news when someone is readmitted.

House call

The house is in what one might call an up-and-coming suburb across the river. Gentrification is happening at a rapid pace all around here, and fairly humble homes that could be had for a reasonable price just a few years ago now sell for unreasonably large sums. Julia and I spoke only rarely about our lives beyond the hospital, or the lives we led prior to the hospital. What was happening in the here-and-now was too pressing. But Julia frequently said she missed her home, and her things.

The hallway is full of oxygen tanks; some are empty, some are full.

'Sorry about all the tanks,' Tom says. 'We just had a delivery. You just ring up and they deliver them …' he says incredulously.

I haven't seen Julia for several weeks, and I am pleased to see her looking relatively well. She wants to know if I like the colour of the walls, and I do. The lounge room is furnished in a minimal retro style, but the feeling is homely. There is good coffee and the promised special cakes. As Tom busies himself with plates and forks, Daisy and Julia are in the middle of a conversation about her teacher.

'I hate him,' Daisy says matter-of-factly. She is avoiding looking at me or acknowledging my presence in any way.

'Why?' Julia wants to know.

'Because he *patronises* me.' She says it with the gusto of someone who has recently discovered what the word means and why it is not OK for someone to do it to you.

After cake, Julia requests that we be left alone so we can have a private conversation.

This is why I'm here. I am not just visiting a friend. I am here because ... Why am I here? Perhaps I am here for a conversation about how to broach the topic that you're going to die, sooner rather than later—much sooner—with your eleven-year-old child, a bright one who doesn't like being patronised.

'So have you had the conversation?'

'Kind of ...'

'What does that mean?' I am gentle but firm, and forthright. No need to beat around the bush.

'Tom says that she never asks him about Mum any more. She always used to ask what was happening with Mum ...'

'Do you think she may be worried about what the news could be?'

'The conversation we had a long time ago, when we ... when I ... was first diagnosed went along the lines of "some people get better from this disease and some die," and she seems to have gone with "some people get better" rather than "some people die ..."'

'What if she is just not saying anything about her fears? That would be my worry,' I say. 'What if she knows or suspects that things are not good?'

We are silent now. Outside, in the garden, people are talking.

'What if you, or Tom, were to say to her, "I've noticed you are no longer asking about me … about your mum …"'

I am mindful of my interaction with Kylie a few weeks ago. *Am I here as Julia's pastoral worker, or as her friend?* We haven't discussed this. I am here on my day off. I am not being paid—but I am not paid anyway. I am not here in any official or professional capacity. I am here as a fellow human being.

'Do you think we could go with, "What if I don't get better?"' Julia asks.

She is teary now. A box of tissues is nearby; I reach for them and hand them to her. It's a gesture we both remember well from another time and place.

'Here we go …' she half-smiles apologetically through the tears.

'It's OK,' I say, even though it doesn't need saying.

The timing is crucial because time works so differently for a child. Are we talking a year or more? A year is such an unbelievably long time for someone who is twelve.

'Maybe the point at which you think or feel you've got less than a year, is that the time … ?'

In fact, Julia doesn't have a year. She has a lot less than that. But we don't know that. Not yet.

She changes the topic. We talk about lots of things—I forget what, exactly. We're like two friends who haven't seen each other for a while. We eat our cake and drink our coffee. And then she says, 'I wouldn't have made it without you,' and she reaches over for my hand.

We remember this from the hospital, too. I want to give her a hug, but she is sitting in a special chair, and she has her oxygen tube that is supposed to go into her nose, but she holds it in her hand and puts it into her mouth between sentences.

'Some people have a living wake,' I say.

She likes that idea.

'I've decided there will be a gathering ... and a tree planting, but no body and no ashes.'

And this is when she asks me if I'd be prepared to give the eulogy. 'If ... if you wanted to, if you felt able to ...' she says hesitantly.

It is as if time stands still. I had no idea she was going to ask me this. I can't speak. I have no words.

'But maybe you're too busy ...'

'I ...' I swallow. 'I ... would be honoured.'

She is crying, and she can barely get a word out.

'Really?'

'Yes. Of course. Absolutely. Thank you for asking me!'

I am just mouthing the words. I can't get any volume out of my voice box, which is busy helping to push the tears down.

'Thank you!'

'No, really, it's me who should be thanking you.'

And now I let them come, the tears that have been wanting to come — and we sit together like that for a while. A person is dying. The person sitting there with her is thinking about a different time, a time when, if people ask, we will say *Julia is dead*.

But that is not now. This is a sparkling, beautiful Sunday afternoon. I stay for another hour or more, and we talk about books and music and films. She tells me that my name reminds her of a European film director. She likes Wim Wenders, and *Wings of Desire* is her favourite, with *Paris, Texas* a close second.

'It's way too long …'

'How can you say that!?'

'Come to think of it, they're both too long. That scene with Natassja Kinski … the monologue in the booth? Where he is just sitting there, going on and on …'

She looks annoyed now.

'I prefer his earlier films …' I say. '*The Goalkeeper's Fear of the Penalty*—have you seen that?'

She hasn't seen it. She will never see it. And then she looks absolutely exhausted all of a sudden, and it's time for me to go. I don't ask the question that I have had in the back of my mind—on the tip of my tongue even—about forgiving the mother. *You're still working on forgiving your mother, aren't you? Because someone else, too, is going to have to forgive her mother. Daisy will have to forgive you … for dying.*

But it just isn't the right time. Maybe there is no right time. Maybe I just lack the courage to ask it. Maybe next time … if there is a next time.

A reason to believe

In the Middle Ages you would have had no choice but to believe in God—and in any case, you would have been too frightened not to—but today's believers, or the ones I speak to about it in the hospital, have all either seen God or they have had some kind of other personal direct experience of His presence. I am surprised by this. I thought you just … you know … had to believe, or else it wouldn't be called faith.

That's what the Bishop of Stepney told me.

You could argue until you're blue in the face that it was an illusion, a trick of the light, a schism of the optical nerve, but no amount of rational argument can make someone stop believing what they've seen with their own eyes or experienced in some way, like the ghost my grandmother saw as a young girl. And if they want to believe, and life is easier in many ways for believers than non-believers, they'll believe it. Ask any magician.

And that's why it's said that there are no atheists in a foxhole, implying that people will choose to believe in God when they are in serious trouble. But I spent three years in a foxhole, on and off, and I found many atheists there. And these are my people. They are my constituents, as it were; this is my congregation. But the irony is this: it's much more difficult for a pastoral worker to get to the non-believers than the believers. The believers are ready, willing, and able to be consoled, to be comforted, but the committed atheists know, or think they know, that consolation is done by Christians, or religious types—and when you introduce yourself as a pastoral worker, they don't want a bar of it. It's like introducing yourself to a staunch Labor voter as the local candidate for the Liberal Party. In the hospital and out of it, as soon as they get an inkling that someone is a Christian, the non-believers will do whatever they can to avoid having to speak with them.

How do I know this? *It is what I'd been doing most of my life!*

It's enough to make me nostalgic for my job at the other hospital, where I went around the wards with the shop trolley.

Most people who are well enough don't mind having a chat if you're selling newspapers and chocolate. All you need for that job is a friendly face.

When I was an artist, many people found me scary, even though I am weedy and average-looking. And I didn't mind that. But when I gave up art and decided I wanted to work with real people, I had to lose the punk scowl I'd perfected over many years. I bought new, friendlier spectacles. But the downside of being the volunteer with the shop trolley is that you are not allowed to talk to people about what it means to be a human being, or what it means to die—and that, it seems, is my calling—if it is a calling, which is what my supervisor says, but then he is a man of the cloth. And I'm not sure I believe in a calling.

So what is it?

I want to say, 'I'm an existential detective!' as in *I Heart Huckabees*, and I tried to get the hospital to put me on as a secular chaplain. When I started, I thought my main customers would be the non-religious patients, but now I'm doing it, I realise it doesn't matter. Everyone in this foxhole is human, and if they need another human to sit with them, I am here for them.

More than 30 per cent of people admitted to the foxhole tick the 'None' box in the section on the form where it asks for your religion. And as soon as I've said, 'I'm a pastoral worker,' some of them say, 'Not interested, thanks'—as if I am a Mormon pastor calling at their house on a Sunday morning. Or they just say, 'I don't want to talk to you.'

Many pastoral encounters begin with the simplest of questions, 'How are you?' It is an opportunity for them to tell me as much or as little of their story as they want to at that moment. Sometimes it works. Sometimes, before they know it, they are telling me the story of their lives, and/or their disease, and their hopes and fears for the future. They're not worried about who I am. They're just happy that I am here, that there is someone to tell their story to. Or people respond with, 'Fine. And who are you?'

During the second half of the year I spend training as a clinical pastoral worker, I become much better at reading when someone is about to tell me to go away. And as they are saying it, I already have my mouth open to tell them I'm a non-believer, and this leads to many deep and meaningful conversations. But it's not always possible, it's not always necessary, and it's not always desirable.

Humour is another useful thing to have in your pastoral toolkit. I learned that early on, one day on my way to morning tea. I was walking past the bed of a man who had previously declined pastoral care. I thought the way he looked at me was not unfriendly, and I'd already realised that sometimes people change their minds because they cannot help but overhear your conversation with someone else in their room, and come to the realisation you're not a god-botherer.

On a whim, I pretended I'd forgotten and said, 'Hello, I'm the pastoral worker on this ward. My name is Joha … Oh, wait. You don't want to talk to me, do you?'

'No,' he said sharply.

'Is it because I'm ugly?'

He couldn't help himself, and laughed, and neither could some of the other people witnessing the encounter. A nurse told me later that this was the first time anyone had seen him laugh since he'd been admitted, and it turned out to be the start of a friendly relationship.

Other times, I am happy to play the straight man. Like with Lawrence, a wiry man in his seventies who had just been diagnosed with lung cancer. He was sitting on the extreme edge of his bed, and glared at me when I introduced myself and asked if he wanted to have a chat.

'Not with a pastoral worker!'

'Don't you like pastoral workers?'

'Now you're trying to have a chat and, like I told you, I don't want to have a chat!' But he smiled, despite himself.

As I walked away, I imagined Lawrence saying to the person in the next bed, 'I got that pastoral worker!'

The ball is round

Johan Cruijff is often said to be the greatest footballer who ever lived, and, at the time of writing, he is still alive — but only just. He was famous for lighting up a cigarette during a break in training, but now he has lung cancer. I saw him play once in Utrecht when my team, DOS, lost 1–7 against Cruijff's Ajax from Amsterdam. Oh how we cheered when DOS finally scored! Cruijff is almost as famous for his Zen-like aphorisms as for his silky ball skills. 'The ball is round', he said once, after an unexpected defeat — in other words, anything can happen in a game of football. Another gem was, 'There's only one moment in which you can arrive on time. If you're not there, you're either too early or too late.' Both are more than apt when it comes to pastoral work.

In Australian Rules football, the ball is not round, as in soccer, but oval, which makes it even more unpredictible —like a football game, there's no way of knowing where a conversation with a person who has cancer will go. Sometimes all someone wants to talk about is football, which is fine with me. I'm always happy to talk football of any variety, except with Collingwood supporters.

One minute you can be talking about the likelihood of the Bulldogs ever winning another flag and the next minute, James, who has been a one-eyed supporter since they last won in 1956, is in tears as he realises he won't live long enough to see them win again.

I go and have a chat with George, an affable Englishman. He is pale as a ghost, but when I ask him how he is, he says he feels fine. I noticed him reading the *Age,* which is usually a good sign. George asks about the work I do, which gives me an opportunity to mark out the territory I cover in my conversations with patients—politics, football, movies, books, the meaning of life, what it means to have cancer. You name it, we can talk about it—and any conversation about anything can turn into a conversation about the meaning of life or what it means to die.

We don't talk much about the latter, but George tells me that the prime minister of the day, Tony Abbott, wanted to be a priest until he found out how long it would take to get to be Pope, and then he decided to go into politics instead. We laugh heartily, but George swears it's true.

He's a Saints fan. Hardly anyone barracks for the Saints, and George is the only person I've ever met who does, except a bloke I used to know years ago — a New Zealander called Ian, who decided to go for them when he came to Australia and needed a team. He chose them because they were the worst team in the league, so that doesn't really count.

In the room next to George is Paul, 25, equally pale and weak from his stem-cell transplant, but very curious. He asks me lots of questions, but gives very little away about himself. After a while, I manage to get out of him that he is a plumber.

'Oh. Good money! Interesting work?'

'Ah, digging trenches, mainly.'

'OK. Whereabouts?'

'Werribee.'

I've always liked the name of that town. 'Been there long?'

'All me life.'

Well, that's not very long!

The hospital is a lonely place for young people. Everyone thinks it is unfair they got cancer so young. I wonder at what age it does become fair. It's not twenty-five — that's for sure.

It's when we get to talking about football that Paul gets going, and then it's hard to get out of the door. When he says he goes for the Magpies, I say, 'OK, well, it's been nice talking to you, but …' and we both laugh. 'I barrack for the Tigers,' I tell him.

Almost everyone hates the Magpies, but most people have a soft spot for the Tigers.

In a different bed on the same ward is another Collingwood fan, Ron, but he's 81. A useful ruckman in his day, he played for seventeen years all over Victoria, but he was 'no good in front of goals, and not fast enough to play football at the elite level'.

Lovely old fellow. Sharp as a tack. *Is it fair at his age?*

It's the end of a long day when Julia is readmitted. I'm just packing up. My mobile rings. I rifle through my bag to find it. It says 'Julia', but it's Tom's voice that says, 'We're in an ambulance on the way to the hospital. Julia asked me to ring you. Are you around?'

'I'll come down.'

I get there as they're taking her out of the ambulance. When she sees me, she just says, 'I'm fucked.'

I take her hand. It's clammy and hot. There is a grim determination in the movements of the ambos, and I can't hold on to her. There is confusion, hustle and bustle, and urgency. She looks around for me — she can't see where I am in relation to the stretcher as we're walking along. When she catches my eye, she says, 'This is the last bit …'

I can't think of anything to say. There is nothing anyone could say. There is nothing to be said.

You're never more of an object than when you are a sick person being transported in a hurry. Everyone is doing their best, I can only presume, but they are clumsy. As they are moving her from the stretcher, they bang her beautiful head on the side of the bed — not once, but twice. She cries out. I try to console her, and then I try to console Tom. I am sweating. I have to go out for a breather. I try to console the nurse she was rude to.

I go back in and sit by the bed for a while. Julia says a couple of odd things that don't make sense. She says a couple of things that do make sense, too. She thanks me for visiting her at home, and says that the conversation we had about Daisy was useful.

The doctors arrive, and I leave, promising to return in the

morning. I walk home. I am sad, sad, sad. King Crimson comes to the rescue. In 1974, at Asbury Park, Fripp takes an entirely different approach to the guitar solo in *Easy Money*. It is at once delicate and threatening. And then all hell breaks loose.

Wednesday

Julia is in no state to talk this morning. When I go back in the afternoon, she is better.

'I don't want to have a funeral.'

'You don't have to have a funeral.'

'Really?'

'No.'

She looks relieved. 'Oh?'

'When you're dead, they can just come and get your body and cremate it, or bury it … Do you want to be buried or cremated …?'

'Cremated.'

'… without anyone having to be there.'

'That's what I want.'

'But you can't stop people wanting to get together and acknowledge the fact that you're dead, and remember you and console each other.'

She ponders that for a while.

'I guess not. But I don't want it to be in a church, and I don't want to have a priest there.'

'Well, you better tell Tom.'

'I will. I just wanted to know what's possible.'

'Everything is possible, you know that.'

She smiles her wan smile. Something about her reminds me of someone I knew a long time ago. Maybe that's why I feel compelled to spend all this time with her. Maybe it isn't even about Julia. Maybe it is about her. Or maybe it is about Daisy. Her mother is about to disappear. Her daughter may be only twelve, but she can see it happening in front of her eyes.

Thursday

I go straight to Julia when I get to the hospital. I spend an hour with her. It's becoming increasingly difficult for her to get enough oxygen. She takes many short, sharp intakes of oxygen from the tube that is meant to go into her nose. When she's talking, she takes it out and puts it into her mouth, and when she gets exasperated, which is frequently, she takes it out of her mouth for a few seconds so she can swear more effectively.

I tell her I can see how much Tom loves her, and she says, 'I know. But why? Why? I don't understand it.'

I move my mouth close to her ear and say very quietly, 'Because you're fucking amazing?'

She takes the tube out of her mouth and scoffs a little, but without much conviction.

She must know she's fucking amazing.

She tells me again how angry and uninterested Daisy seems, and I say, 'I think you've just got to tell her that you are sorry … And that you would make the choice to still be there for her … *if* you had a choice.'

We both cry.

'This will be the hardest thing you have done in your entire life. Are you ready?'

She just looks at me. I think I can see fear in her eyes. But I don't think it is being dead that she is afraid of.

After seeing Julia, I run around trying to catch up with the doctor whom Tom had 'words' with this morning. Tom is not happy with the treatment Julia is getting. He told the doctor he is incompetent. That never goes down well, but especially not with doctors. The doctor has rung and left a message asking to see me to get some background on the 'case.'

I finally locate the doctor. He is wearing a nice three-piece suit. He is just leaving the hospital, and doesn't really have time to talk now. I walk along with him and I say, 'Tom is losing his wife and the mother of his daughter. He is angry, and he is sad.'

That is about all you'd need to know about the 'case' at this stage.

Friday

Outside it's another grey day. It is cold and threatening to rain. Inside, Julia is unconscious. Her breathing is laboured. The brothers, her mother, the husband, and daughter are all in and out of there. I spend several hours with them. At one point I am alone in the room with Julia and her daughter.

I say to Daisy, 'There is every chance that she can still hear you. Is there something you need to say to her?'

She shakes her head.

'Have you said goodbye to her?'

'Yes.'

She's a good actor. It's as if she doesn't have a care in the world. Julia's mother produces a bag of sweets from her bag and hands it to Daisy. She eats several, one after the other—a green one, then a yellow one, and then an orange one. She has a red pompom in her hair, and owl clip-on earrings.

'I have to eat sweets to calm myself down,' she says—and everyone laughs nervously.

In a different room on the same ward, just across the corridor, the shoe is on the other foot. A mother is watching her child writhing in pain. She is weeping bitterly. She says to me, 'We buried the other one twenty-eight years ago. He was a year older. They were like twins.'

The room is full of people: the brothers and sisters, their husbands and wives, his mother and father, his children and his wife. They are mostly crying and watching in horror. There is nothing they can do for him.

The nurse in charge is tearing her hair out. Her voice is choked with emotion. She tells me, 'This sometimes happens. There is just nothing we can do for him. I mean, we are giving him enough hydromorphone to kill him.'

I watch him hug each of his daughters in turn and cry. There are three of them. One of them is in her early twenties, and she keeps saying, 'It's all right, Dad. You're fine. It's OK.'

By saying it, she is hoping to make it so. It's the only thing she can think of. I wish she would say, 'I can hear and see that it's not all right, Dad, and it's not OK.'

Rita, his wife, is saying to him, 'Remember how you used to carry them when they were babies? How we used to take them to the park?'

She is recalling all kinds of memories of their children for him as he cries and yells out in pain and struggles for breath, struggles to remain a human being. In the room across the corridor, being able to be a human being is becoming more and more difficult for Julia, too.

Sunday

Julia has been unconscious since Friday, and her pain medication has been increased. Tom has not had much sleep since Julia began deteriorating, and he needs to debrief about everything that has happened since I was in the hospital on Friday. He believes Julia is close to the end of her life. We discuss funeral arrangements and ideas for a memorial service. One of her brothers is collecting photographs for a slide show. There will be a projector and a screen. Tom asks me if I would be prepared speak at the service.

'It would be an honour.'

There is a certain point when we start talking about the person in the past tense — even though they are still there with us, if only barely, in the room, and still breathing, albeit with great difficulty. And every one of those breaths could be the last.

I am at home when Julia's brother Robert rings, just after dinner, to say Julia has died. I ask about the end.

'She became quite uncomfortable right at the end,' he tells me, 'but it didn't last long.'

I offer my condolences. He says they don't need anything, and there's no need for me to come back to the hospital. I should have said, *I'll come anyway. I want to come.* But they might want some privacy. And the brothers don't really know me from Adam.

An hour later, there's a call from Ward 4, asking if I can come back to the hospital and see a patient who is distressed. On the way, I go into Julia's room to ... do what ... ? to say goodbye? to view the body? When my father died, I didn't want to view the body. As a teenager, I'd seen what was left of a man who'd jumped in front of a train, and I never wanted to see a body again—least of all the body of my father. Several family members tried to persuade me that it would be good to 'have a viewing.' He looks good, they told me. It might help with closure, whatever that is. But I steadfastly refused.

I don't know. It had been such a long ... shall we call it a process? We talked about it so often, and now it is here. Now it is a fact. There she is. Or what remains of her.

The family is gone. I stand there alone for a few minutes with what remains of my almost-friend. But she's not there any more. She wasn't really *there* yesterday either. Her body is still, now. The urgent gasping for breath has stopped. You wouldn't say it was peaceful, because it is not. It is nothing. But there is none of the noise that was always present at the end. No drip, no monitors, no oxygen flowing. All the tubing is gone. And so is her discomfort, her suffering. It's so strange to see her now, so literally drained of life, almost grey, a shell, like something an insect leaves behind after metamorphosis.

Monday

I rang Tom this morning to see how he was. Daisy answered the phone, but I didn't have the presence of mind to try to talk to her about what had happened. And I wouldn't be keen to talk about something so delicate and raw with someone so young, unless I could look her in the eye. I was lost for words with Tom, too, but I let him know that I was there for him, and that if he wanted to have a coffee, to give me a call.

'I might just take you up on that.'

'I hope you do.'

And that's where I had to leave it. I did have something real and good for him: I wanted to say that when a person dies, the connection remains alive. You are still connected to what the dead person thought and said. But, again, the telephone does not seem the right medium through which to transmit such a message.

It came to me during the night. I felt a quietness around Julia's death. *It is as if she is part of me now.* It is as if when someone dies, it is the body that's left behind, but all the time we spent together, the feelings, the doubt, the fear she communicated to me, but also her courage, her defiance—and the conversations we had—have become part of me. She is not *really* dead. She has lost her ability to be. She no longer *is* a human being. But something continues to live, in a different form. I remain connected to her, and what she was to me, she is still. There is a huge hole there, of course there is—a palpable absence. This feeling does not fill that. Each day, each morning, I'll feel it, and when I go to bed at night. But she is still there, and I could talk to her if I wanted to. All of her thoughts and feelings and experiences have become part of the collective unconscious—and although I can't access them directly, they are not lost.

Julia is dead, but Sidonie is worried about the Muslims.

'They tell them to have at least five children, and we're only having one or two. And they don't do as they're told!'

'The children or the Muslims?'

'Eh?'

There's no point pursuing it—and there's not much else to say. She's doesn't want to talk or think about what is happening to her, or what the future holds.

'Just taking it one day at a time …' Sidonie says, waving her hand. And she's not taking an active interest in her treatment.

'Just leave it in the hands of the experts …'

And that's exactly how they like it.

Mary, in the bed next to Sidonie, tells me a series of random facts about her life. She is a transcendental meditator. She tells me the doctor said she has an interesting cancer. *Heaven forbid that you'd have a boring cancer.* She is about to sponsor a different child.

'You only do it for seven years, and then it stops. Maybe it's when they're older that the money stops?'

'That seems a bit arbitrary. Don't older children and young adults have needs?'

I tell Mary I used to send $100 a month to a Rwandan child and her grandmother when I was still earning. The money I sent was spent on clothes for the child and schoolbooks, and sometimes seed or chickens for their little bit of land. There was no money for the child to go to school. That's what it said on the website. I guess they didn't need a hundred dollars worth of clothes and schoolbooks every month. But when I stopped earning, I had to stop sending.

I knew a heroin addict in Newcastle once who sponsored a child. Now that's commitment. A junkie usually only has one thing and one thing only that they are truly committed to finding the money for. But Dave was unusual in a number of other ways, too. But I digress. Mary asks about my morning. That, too, is unusual. I tell her about the joy of someone who is allowed to leave the hospital.

Tuesday

Julia is dead, and I wonder if she lived long enough to begin to forgive her mother for being cruel. I am grateful I lived long enough to forgive my mother. I hope she doesn't read this. She'll probably say, 'Have you gone insane? What are you talking about?' I could remind her of a few things. She's probably forgotten. Even today, when she tells a story about something naïve I said in all seriousness when I was a child, and everyone laughs, I weep inside. I feel every bit as small and insignificant as I did then.

Forgetting just *happens*. And it's endless. Forgetting. Remembering. Forgetting again. You think you've forgotten something, and then you remember it again. But forgiving is work, and it's ongoing. It's a process that is infinite and infinitely demanding. It is work you have do in your own psyche. You can say it quietly, or just think it. And it is never too late. But the best time to begin is always now. *I forgive you.* It does require you to be alive, though. Once you're dead, it doesn't matter anymore — or, it matters, but it's too late. You missed the boat. So it goes.

The spirit of things

Julia is dead, and there is a new ward clerk in the intensive-care unit. Her name is Kerry. I think that's what she said. She wears a lot of make-up, and looks like a frightened rabbit. There is a new nurse in charge, too — Clarissa. She exudes competence, but also compassion. Clarissa suggests I go and talk to Harold, who has only had sporadic visitors and is having a really difficult time. He has advanced lung cancer. She explains it won't be easy to communicate because he is intubated and wearing a pressurised oxygen mask.

She says, 'It might be too difficult,' and looks at me as if she's giving me an out, or like she's expecting me to say, 'Ah, yes, that would be too difficult.'

But I thank her for the referral, and go and introduce myself to Harold, who has what sounds like a Scottish accent. It's hard to tell from underneath the mask. I can understand that he's not happy and that he's frustrated, but he says a number of things that I don't understand, despite straining my ears and my brain.

I point at his little radio. 'At least you've got the radio, Harold.'

He nods.

'What sort of things do you like to listen to? The news?'

He nods.

'Football?'

He shakes his head.

'You don't like football?!'

He shakes again. The many tubes going into and coming out of his head make shaking it difficult, but spectacular. He becomes very frustrated and visibly angry because I keep asking him to repeat what he is saying. I am breaking into a sweat. He is very insistent.

'John Cleary, *The Religion Report*. Rachel Kohn, *The Spirit of Things*!'

Finally, I get it. 'AAAH! JOHN CLEARY! THE RELIGION REPORT!!'

He nods vigorously.

'THE SPIRIT OF THINGS!! RACHEL KOHN!!!'

But he's been trying so hard, he is very red in the face. An alarm goes off. Clarissa comes over and tells me I will have to go. Harold is doing too much talking.

'Breathing comes first,' she says, and looks at me sternly.

I feel sad.

'I have to go, I am sorry,' I tell him. I take his hand.

'Take care, mate.'

I give him my card. He thanks me. He is just grateful for

the interaction, I think. There was some mention of a partner who travels a lot for work. He doesn't come very often. *Where is he?*

For many people, it's just too much. They simply can't cope with being in the same room as their loved one when they're suffering so much, and it's so hard to have a conversation. It's OK. That's just how it is. *And that is why I am here.*

I see him again a few days later. He's been extubated. I don't think he remembers me.

'Hello, Harold!'

'Hello.'

'Last week we were talking about *The Religion Report* and *The Spirit of Things* ...' I remind him.

He smiles. 'Ah. You remember!'

My favourite patient in the hospital today is Nina, a splendid woman in her seventies who welcomes me enthusiastically into her room. She is packing up. She's finally going home after four weeks in the hospital. She is eager to have a conversation. We cover a lot of ground very quickly, and she talks easily about the love of her life, her husband, John. She tells me the story of how they met. It was back when you'd meet your future wife or husband at the yearly dance in the local hall.

'Everyone would come from all around. It was a big deal!' She smiles.

'He wanted to dance with me, but I wasn't keen.'

'Why not?'

'He had a reputation!'

'Oh, I see!' We laugh. 'But then you changed your mind.'

'I did … I certainly did!' she says tenderly. 'Here he is now!'

A large man with beige trousers and a jovial, red face enters the room.

'Are you ready, darl?' he booms. 'Oh, who is this?'

'I'm just the p …'

'This is Yo-han … the pastoral worker,' Nina interrupts. 'Am I pronouncing your name right?'

'Close enough,' I smile.

John is already busying himself with the suitcases.

'Where did all this stuff come from!' he says in mock exasperation, but he's smiling.

'I'm so glad that I got to meet you, Nina. Good luck.'

I hold out my hand, but she wants a hug. We hug.

'And me you, darling. Thanks very much'

I didn't do anything!

Two dying men

There are two dying men. I comfort them in the same hour, and it seems to come easily to me now, comforting the dying. What I mean is, I walk into the hospital as an ordinary person, but somehow I become extraordinary. I am like Batman. It is as if it has nothing to do with me. It just happens. I am talking to the nurse in charge. I am ordinary. Then, as I walk towards the patient's room, it happens—the transformation.

In the room is Jim. He is in a bad way. I tell him who I am, and he says, 'I'm Jim.'

And now I am full of compassion and, yes, I think it is pity that I am feeling. I offer my hand. He takes it with an edge of desperation. It is as if he is trying to draw some strength from me. I ask him how he is doing.

'No good. No good.'

That's all he can get out. It is so hard for him to breathe.

'He is very uncomfortable,' I say to the nurse in charge. What I mean is: *He is suffering.* And his bed is dirty.

The other one is Vince. He … or maybe it was his brother … requested a visit from a priest, and I accompany the priest when he arrives. Vince has a simple-enough question for the priest, and it is this: 'Why?'

He's never done anything wrong, and he used to go church every day, seven days a week.

'And now this!' he says to the priest. But the priest says nothing. He doesn't seem keen to offer an explanation.

I say to Vince, 'We don't know. Maybe God can tell you why, when you get to heaven.'

He is drifting in and out of consciousness. I stroke his head.

The priest is keen to get going. 'Shall I come back later?' he says to Vince.

Vince opens his eyes. He looks at the priest as if he is seeing him for the first time.

'Wha … ?'

The priest says, 'I can give communion.'

He taps his pocket like a drug dealer. I don't think Vince can understand a word the priest is saying, either because of the drugs he's on or because the priest, who is Nigerian, speaks with a heavy accent.

'I have communion with me,' he says again.

I say, 'Vince, would you like to have a blessing? Would you like to take communion?'

Of course he does. How could you say no?

The priest is pleased. Finally he can be of use. He says, 'This is the body of Christ.'

And Vince responds in the expected way. He takes the offered bread and puts it in his mouth. He makes the sign of the cross. I always like this moment of silence when the deed is done and we just stand around. Vince masticates with folded hands. Vince swallows and says, 'I am not afraid.'

A God moment

Julia is dead. Last night I dreamed there was a dying horse in my garden.

The believers have a term for events or experiences they interpret as a sign that there is a God and that he has a plan for them. It may be an epiphany or some kind of mini-revelation—like the burning bush perhaps, or a dream. They call it 'a God moment.' And they talk in terms of needing to protect that experience. I guess for them it's evidence in their struggle against doubt and unbelief.

It is an irony worthy of an omnipotent supernatural being that the same thing applies to us non-believers—except what we have to protect ourselves against is getting sucked into believing it's a sign that there is a creator with a master plan, and instead continue with the demanding work of interpreting signs in a non-religious way.

I like to say 'non-believer' rather than 'atheist' because I have too much doubt to believe in atheism. What *we* must resist, those of us who are non-believers, is nihilism. We must be radical optimists and believe in … what … ? Lots of things … possibilities … humans … reason … ethics … equality … choices … *freedom*! All of these and many other mysterious things are interesting to us. What is not interesting to us is people demanding that we believe in some kind of supernatural fat controller. And we accept being 'large with not-knowing,' as Xander puts it in *Buffy the Vampire Slayer*.

And I have no idea why I dreamt about a dying horse.

The mummy's boy

Julia is dead. I spend an hour with an elderly lady called Luisa. She is the mother of a young woman on my ward called Cathy. I met Cathy yesterday, and we had some significant time together. She was quite forthright in her conversation with me, and she mentioned her anxious mother. I was committed to staying there for as long as it took. It took a considerable amount of time. It ended with her hugging me.

After lunch today, when I went up to check on her, Cathy welcomed me by looking around the room and announcing, 'Here is the man who managed to calm me down …' And she put out her arms for another hug.

She asked me if I could have a chat with her mother, and I do. I am similarly calm and confident with her, but I don't manage to work the same miracle with Luisa that I somehow did with her daughter. She keeps checking to see if a doctor or a nurse is coming, and then she looks at me as if she's not convinced.

And then there is Tracy. She is the mother of two children, both of whom killed themselves four weeks apart. 'Lost to suicide,' is how she puts it. Rebecca, 21, was first, and her brother went four weeks later.

'He took it hard. He *loved* his big sister!'

And it was in this four-week period that she was diagnosed with cancer. She tells me all this with a quiet detachment. She tells me about her ex-husband, the father of the children: 'He was a mummy's boy!'

I have to laugh.

'He couldn't even buy an Esky without checking with his mother,' she says bitterly.

My mother instilled in me at an early age the idea that I owed her a great debt of gratitude for all the sacrifices she'd made on my behalf. As the decades rolled by, I got the feeling that no matter what I did, I would never be able to repay her. And then one day—I must have been in my forties—it suddenly dawned on me that, all along, she had just been doing what she felt she had to do. And I was a child. I had no choice in the matter. Respecting your elders is fair enough; I'm not opposed to it. But the adults would do themselves and everyone else a great favour if they resisted the temptation to mock us because we're young and naïve. Because we will come back to haunt you when you are old and feeble and we are all grown up with fully functioning brains.

From what I've seen of Tracy's new husband-to-be, he

doesn't seem much of an improvement on the old one, but I can't say anything. She is 51, she has cancer, and she needs someone.

Free coffee

I've arranged to have coffee with Richard, the pastoral worker at the hospice where Julia was for a few weeks after she left the hospital for the first time. He invited me to come for a visit. On the phone he said, 'She spoke of you often.'

He is a portly Christian with a beard, and friendly enough, but I don't warm to him. He seems a bit random. He doesn't make a lot of eye contact. He strikes me as a troubled man. And it's as if he's constantly looking around to see if someone more interesting is coming. *I am kind of getting the feeling he's checking me out … as if I am a potential rival. God knows why. Maybe he's ambitious.*

Richard is enthusiastically telling me about the coffee.

'It is free!'

It comes from a machine that puts sugar into your coffee by default.

'If you don't want sugar, you have to press 'SUGAR' before you press the 'COFFEE' button to make the coffee,' he explains after I've already pressed 'COFFEE'.

There is a moral in there somewhere, but I can't for the life of me figure out what it is.

Richard takes me on a tour of the facility. There is an awful lot of grey in the hospice — grey walls, grey floors, grey curtains. In the Day Hospice, there is homemade cake on offer, so I have a piece. It has raw cake mix in the centre.

I see a couple of old people in their beds in passing. They look sad and lonely. But Richard doesn't introduce me to any patients, only to staff. They all look like they'd rather be somewhere else. This half-baked environment would have depressed the bejesus out of Julia. How humiliating for an atheist—not to mention someone who was as particular about coffee and cake as she was—to have had to check into a Catholic hospice. Although there are some beds in the hospital that are nominally palliative beds, the government doesn't fund hospices; so if it's taking you a while to die, you end up sharing the end of your life with Christian references and artefacts.

Richard asks why I didn't go into art therapy.

'Because it's all smoke and mirrors.'

He asks how the way I work with patients differs from a psychologist, if I am not religious. As if by way of explanation, he adds, 'You *look* like a psychologist.'

I don't know how to take that. I am wearing my good jacket for the occasion. Richard looks like someone who is going to Bunnings to buy planks.

'Because I don't pathologise or problematise?'

There is a lot of work to do. Many believers seem to find it difficult to imagine what non-believers do and/or think. It must be strange for them.

Richard tells me about an art project that's just been installed in one of the other hospitals in town: it's called the Disambiguation Room. It's supposed to have a therapeutic effect.

What's wrong with ambiguity? Perhaps that's why people need

*religion. Because they're uncomfortable with ambiguity? But then
Judaism is all ambiguity! Maybe that's why they had to invent
Jesus Christ ...*

Richard wants to know what I do with people who have a
theological problem.

'You mean like "Why did God give me cancer?"'

'For instance.'

'Yeah. That's a tough one! The secular version of it is not
that different: "Why did I get cancer?" I generally let that
go through to the keeper. Although I did say to someone
once, "Why do *you* think God gave you cancer?" after he
had essentially confessed to having been a sex tourist. But he
didn't make the connection. He thought he'd been helping
the local economy. However, if the theological question is
about the meaning of a text, I can offer my reading of it. I'm
happy to do that ...'

Richard looks bored.

'Say if the question was, "What do you think Jesus meant
when he said so and so?" I can say what I think. But otherwise
I would have to refer them to someone from their particular
religious tradition. Do you think that's a problem?'

Richard looks thoughtful, but he doesn't say anything.
Does he think I'm dangerous?

'How do you, as a Christian, deal with a Buddhist, or a
Muslim, with a theological problem?' I ask Richard.

'They don't really ask me.'

I take this as a joke and I laugh heartily, but Richard looks
at me strangely. He asks why I don't make art anymore.

'Because there are already so many *things* in the world, and
I don't want to add to them.'

He says he feels like that too sometimes, about his paintings.

'You're a painter?'

'Yes. And I've got an exhibition coming up! Have I got your email? I'll send you an invitation.'

Great! A few days later, along with the invitation, he sends me a copy of his Master of Theology thesis. As a former supervisor of Masters theses, I would say it's exceptionally well researched and eloquent. There is obviously a brain in there, but I have no interest at all in painting. I never did—even when I was being paid to seem interested.

The work of mourning

It is nearly spring, but it's still cold and it's been raining, on and off. Large, dark clouds are moving at speed overhead. The sky could open up at any moment. At the gathering to remember Julia, there is an audience of maybe sixty or seventy. Most of them will be wondering who the hell I am and what I am doing here, and there are several who are also anxiously eyeing the clouds.

> Friends and family of Julia, Tom, Daisy—thank you. It is an honour to be invited to speak here. There is so much that I could say and would like to say about the remarkable person that she was and about what Julia taught me about death and dying—but I am mindful of the weather and the fact that many things have already been said, so I will be brief.

I am giving a eulogy today. I'm doing it because she asked me to. It's not the last thing I will do for Julia. She also asked me to 'keep an eye on them'—that is, Tom and Daisy. I will do that, too. I'm not sure how yet, but I'll figure it out, just like I figured out how to do the other things she asked me to do—like being there for a dying woman with a twelve-year-old child in the last three months of her life.

I probably knew Julia for less time than any of you here today. I was just her pastoral worker in the hospital. I say 'just' because it became a private joke between us. Julia would admonish me and say, 'Can we do without the 'just'?'

I want to tell them about how it began, my almost-friendship with Julia, how it began with me sitting there holding the thin hand of a bewildered, frightened woman who was coming to the realisation that she didn't have long to live.

I suspect that when the nurse told her that she would call for the pastoral worker on May the third, which was the day I first met her, Julia was worried. One of the first things she asked me about was my religious affiliation. When I said I'm an atheist, she said, with what I came to think of as her characteristic half-grin, 'Thank God! So am I.' (Pause for laughter?)

Julia taught me a number of fundamentally important things about how to do this work. She made me realise that the bottom line is you have to be prepared to *be there*—that is, if they want you there. If they don't want you there, well, then, what you have to do is even simpler. You have to go away. And almost invariably, what they want you to do will be crystal clear, if you're paying attention.

> I only knew her for three months, but they were the last three months of her life—and during this time, as it became clear that she might not live much longer, we discussed in detail the big questions about the human condition: what it means to live, what it means to be a human being, and what it means to die.

Julia wanted me to be here. Looking around as I am speaking, I can see that what I am saying is connecting with many of the people here, that it is meaningful for them. And they want me to be here. They want someone to talk to them about what it was like for her at the end.

> There were three people that Julia talked about a lot with me in the last three months of her life. Her mother and Tom, of course—and how she came to be with him and what a good man he is. I felt privileged to be able to witness how much he loved her. When I told her this she said, 'But why? I don't understand why!'
>
> And I said, 'Because you are amazing!'

I had toyed with the idea of repeating what I actually said, and I still had not given up entirely on the idea when I was standing there, but in the end I decide to err on the side of caution.

But the person we spent most time talking about was Daisy—and to Daisy, I want to say this:

I said to Julia, 'Perhaps you could write Daisy a letter that she can read when she is 18.' The last time we spoke about it she said she had written half of it. I hope she had time to finish it.

The immensity of Julia's grief of leaving you was not a selfish grief. She grieved, not for herself but because she was so very, very sorry to leave you. She wanted so much to be able to continue to be there for you.

Remember that.

Being there, being a human being when another human is suffering is hard, but it's not brain surgery. Be yourself. Sometimes there is something you can say, and sometimes there is nothing. And right now, what is needed is that I speak these words:

At the end she was in a place where she accepted what was happening to her—which doesn't mean that she was not grieving—because grief and acceptance are not mutually exclusive.

But as you mourn her, remember that, although her body is gone, and she can no longer be present in the same dimensions as us, and the particles that constituted her have been dispersed and will eventually make their way back to the stars from which they came, our connection with her remains alive.

Our connection with her ideas, her words, the things she believed, were important: to live an ethical life, to be committed to doing things well, to respect other human beings and treat them as equals.

As non-believers, like Julia was, proudly, defiantly—as I'm sure many of you gathered here today are—we don't have a god to pray to, or a heaven to go to when we die. We believe not in god but in humans—and all humans must die, that is the reality. We trust not in god but in ourselves and each other. Our work is to think about what it means to be a human being, and this is what Julia did during the last three months of her life.

In some ways, dying is easy. What makes it hard is your love for the people you have to leave behind—her many friends, her mother and brothers, Tom, and above all Daisy—who are mourning her and who will continue to mourn her.

As the French philosopher Jacques Derrida said, 'The work of mourning is never finished.'

And this is the work you must face when you leave here today.

Be brave. Be strong. Be conscious.

As Julia was, and as she would have wanted you to be.

Afterwards there is cake and tea and coffee, or beer and wine for those who want it. I am not usually one to say no to cake, but I am too busy—a dozen or more people want to speak to me, to thank me or tell me that what I'd said was helpful or meaningful. Someone says, 'It was beautiful,' and others remark on one or another detail of what I said.

Oh, what I would have given for such undivided attention

when I was lecturing, or for such an appreciative audience when I was an artist.

One sad-faced woman comes over and, without saying anything, puts her hand on my arm. And then she says, 'I wish you could have been there for my husband. He died last year. We had twenty-four years.'

That's how long they were together. He was the best friend of one of Julia's brothers.

A year ago, almost to the day, I was driving out of the university gates for the last time. This is everything I always wanted 'work' to mean—the kind of work that is also a gift. And this is everything I've always wanted to be and wanted to be able to give. And this is what I always thought I could be and would be able to give. And here and now there is no need or reason for me to be anything more or less than I am, or to give any more or less than I am able to give. It is a moment of supreme happiness in the midst of an immense sadness.

A Clown and a Priest

Life is shit

In the lift, I meet the father of a young man on 10.

'Life is shit,' he says. 'I'm sorry.'

'Don't say sorry! You're perfectly entitled to feel like that!'

He has a lot to say, and it is as if he only has a short time to say it. The words tumble out of him, and he apologises again.

'I'm talking too much …'

'No, you're not. You can talk.'

He calls me 'Father'.

Ah well.

An artist, Christian Boltanski, once said, 'I am a cross between a clown and a priest.'

Maybe what I do now is not so different, actually, from what I was doing before.

Talking of priests, I am surprised how hard it is to get a priest to come to the hospital. I'd always thought they'd be tripping over each other if someone wanted them to come. But I've learned this is not the case. I suppose there are cost-cutting pressures and human-resource-management experts in the church, the same as in any other organisation. There are many phone numbers to try, and messages are left that are not responded to.

The endgame

Warwick is sitting up in his bed in Intensive Care, a Tigers scarf resting on his pillow. Last night's game against the Bombers didn't matter one iota in terms of the finals, but it mattered to Warwick because his life support is being turned off today. His lungs are completely shot. He is in his mid-forties. Things are looking good for the Tigers next year, everyone says, but Warwick won't be there to see it.

I used to tell my students that art is a matter of life and death, and some people say the same thing about football. But here, now, it is not merely metaphorical. When you're hanging on for dear life, something as normal and everyday as football literally becomes a way of not dying.

James was as philosophical about dying as he was about his football team, and in the months that he was wasting away on my ward, his beloved Bulldogs were having one of their worst seasons for a long time.

'They should never have changed their name,' he told me.

I didn't have the heart to remind him that they were just as hopeless when they were still called Footscray.

Last night, Warwick's mate came to the hospital, and they watched the game together, the nurse said. It was the Tigers' second-last game of the season, but it was the last game Warwick will ever see.

I watched the game, too, with one of my oldest friends, Michael, a Bombers fan. After all these years, about the only thing we still have in common is football, and we usually go to the game when our teams play each other. This time, because rain was predicted, he proposed watching it on TV at his house instead of traipsing out to the Melbourne Cricket Ground—but the real reason he didn't want to be there was that his Bombers were a waste of space, and last night they didn't have a hope in hell of beating the Tigers.

Michael's wife, Mercedes, is Mexican. She made empanadas. Michael is proud of his wife's empanadas. We ate them with sour cream and lettuce.

'These are the real deal,' he said, beaming.

They were nice enough, but maybe Mercedes was worried about the sensitivity of my Australian palate. I thought the fillings were a little under-seasoned, as were the Tigers, but they won easily and played well enough, although they were wasteful, kicking many more behinds than goals.

Mercedes has no interest in football, but she was curious and talkative. She asked me many questions—some of them general, almost philosophical, some more specific. None of them seemed to have any relationship to the other, and they didn't follow any recognisable pattern.

'How old is your wife?'

'What time does the game finish?'

'Where did you buy your shoes?'

'Why does Ivan, um, Ma … Murich …?'

'Maric,' Michael said, smiling. She smiled back.

'… have a … what do you call it?'

'A mullet!' I laughed.

She laughed gregariously. 'Yes! A … mullet!'

She pronounced it as if it were a French word for a species of fish: *Moulette*.

'I'm not sure,' I said. 'I think, to begin with, it was ironic. But now it's his tradem …'

As well as jumping from one topic to another without rhyme or reason, she didn't let me finish answering a single question before asking another one.

'What makes for a good cat?'

They have a cat they don't like. He is an anxious boy cat with interesting stripes, who lives mainly outside. When he was sniffing me to find out why I looked like a human but smelled like a cat, I picked him up to say hello, and he was like, *Eh? What's this cat/human doing to me?!* And struggled to get away.

'Umm ... one that sits on your lap and purrs when you pat him?' I offered.

At half-time we stood on the back porch in the cold so that Michael could smoke. I used to smoke, but I gave up years ago, and now I don't really approve of smoking. But I don't have many friends, so I didn't say anything about it — and I tried not to notice my discomfort when I had to breathe in his smoke.

'So life is good?' I said to Michael.

'Yeah ... it's good ...' he mumbled. 'But ... sometimes I get a little bored.'

'Hmmm ... OK. How old are you now?'

'Forty-five.'

'That's a great age,' I said, 'a perfect age.'

He didn't ask me why I thought that, so I didn't tell him.

Driving home, I felt sad.

'Never be bored,' I wanted to say to Michael. 'Every moment is precious, every second, each and every breath. What if this was the last game you ever saw the Bombers play? What if this was the last time you held your boy in your arms and made him laugh?'

How many times have I seen this in the hospital?

And instead of living in Mexico, they live in a house in Melbourne that costs them only three hundred dollars a week. The kids are both cute and free of deformities and mental impairments. I mean, he really should be counting his blessings. But you can't say that to people, or you become an old bore, and they stop inviting you around for authentic empanadas made by a real Mexican on a cold night when you don't want to go the ground to watch the game because its raining and anyway your team has no chance of making the finals. But Warwick would have loved to be there.

And when I come in on Saturday, the bed is empty, but the yellow-and-black balloons and the other decorations are still there, as is his scarf—an old-school home-knitted scarf from the time before football became big business.

Thank God the Tigers won.

Meat

Terry the security guard is a Tigers fan, too, or so he claims. But you can't have a conversation about football with him. His knowledge of football is limited to the headlines on the back page of the *Herald Sun*.

'I see Riewoldt is underperforming again,' he offers.

'That's the other Riewoldt, Terry. Jack kicked a bag!'

Terry is more interested in telling me in great detail about the excellent quality of the meat sold at a butcher shop he's discovered in Ivanhoe. Apparently, the most succulent steaks and perfect sausages can be had from this butcher, but Terry has to take his mum with him when he goes. He raises his eyebrows and says, 'She's Italian ...' as if that should mean something significant to me.

'So there's no truth in the rumour that you're a vegetarian then, Terry?'

He looks hurt.

'None', he says emphatically. 'No chance.'

Mount Kilamanjaro

'Two weeks ago I was halfway up Mount Kilamanjaro,' Magriet is telling me, 'and now I'm in here.'

A South African woman of forty-five, with beautiful teeth and dual nationality, she was healthy, and employed in 'a top management position in the travel industry'.

'Never been in a hospital in my life!'

She quickly arranged to leave the Cape Town hospital where she was diagnosed, and returned to Australia. Visibly relieved to be back in a country where public health-care is free and of the same standard as private care, at least in theory, she says how grateful she is that she was able to get back to Australia for treatment. But what she wants now is answers.

'What's happening to me?' she asks, her eyes widening as she speaks. 'Can they fix it?'

'I'm just the pastoral worker. I don't know. When are you seeing your doctor?'

The next morning in the ward meeting, the charge nurse is

Carla. She is at the start of the second half of a double shift, and she doesn't looks happy about it. She races through the names next to the bed numbers on the big whiteboard in the handover room. Magriet is last on the list.

'She's *riddled* with cancer,' Carla says, 'but she doesn't know it yet.'

'When will she be told?' someone asks.

'Her doctor is away until Tuesday, so we'll ask social work to arrange a family meeting for Tuesday,' Carla says, brusquely.

When someone is given bad news, there is safety in numbers. As many people as possible are present — family and staff. Depending on who the social worker is that's running the meeting, and their view of pastoral care, sometimes they like to have a pastoral worker on hand. The social worker on my ward is Barbara. She always has her hands quite full, and is usually seen hurrying from one place to another carrying a bunch of files, ring binders, and clipboards. In my two months of work on this ward, she has barely acknowledged my existence, and still only does so if I greet her first. I don't blame her, but I don't think she'll be asking me to come to the family meeting.

My chest feels tight. Today is Thursday. I'll see Magriet at least three times between now and Tuesday, unless I try to avoid her. I'm just a pastoral worker. My job is not medical in nature. I attend the daily ward meetings, together with the other allied health staff, in order to be informed and to receive referrals, but we are usually referred to patients only when the staff member believes the patient has 'spiritual' issues, or when they've completely run out of ideas.

As someone who doesn't believe in supernatural beings

or life after death, what I understand by 'spiritual' is different from most people, but almost everyone who has cancer is thinking about what it means to die, and what it means to live. Whether they want to talk about it—with me or with anyone else—is another matter. But I can try.

I know Magriet is dying. But I can't talk to her about that. Not yet.

David's rifle

David says, 'You know … it's a pity.'

'What is?'

'I didn't bring my rifle with me.'

'Oh?!'

'They wouldn't let me take it in the ambulance.'

'Would that be for me—or for you?'

'If you give me the shits, it's for you.'

'Well, here's hoping I don't give you the shits then!'

'Ah well. We all give someone the shits at some point, don't we?'

'I guess so! See you!'

The walking song

Thursday is not my favourite day of the week. It's the day I leave the hospital at lunchtime to go and earn some money.

I was lucky enough to be able to find a job where I can work for four hours and earn enough to pay the rent. I am grateful. Ironically, it's in an educational institution. But I'm not being paid to teach; I'm being paid to fix their computers. On Thursday mornings I work with people whose problem is that they are dying, and in the afternoons I'm working with people whose problem is that their mouse doesn't work.

What made this Thursday worse was that I had an argument with a priest, but it wasn't about the existence of God. I'd left a message for him yesterday, saying, 'There's a patient on 4 who's requested a Catholic priest.' When I saw her on my round this morning, I asked if a priest had come, and she said no. So I rang the priest again. This time he answered, but he wanted to know what the patient wanted.

'She wants to see a priest …!'

'What about?'

'I don't know. Maybe communion … or confession?'

'Well, we don't do communion …'

'OK, so you can tell her that when you visit her.'

'Well, it's the job of pastoral care to find out what the patient wants.'

'Look, what the patient wants is to see a Catholic priest. So that's the message I'm giving to you. But if you don't want to see her, I'll go and tell her that.'

I slammed the phone down.

Today, the priest arrives just as I am leaving the hospital en route to my appointment with a lung specialist. When I had my medical at the beginning of the year, they found something in my blood that they didn't like, and it's taken a good six months to have X-rays done and to get an appointment to see a specialist. It was a nice walk in the park to the doctor. It was very cold, but fresh and good.

I am grateful to be in the hands of a real, old-style gentle doctor who smiles and behaves like a fellow human being, and who is happy to take all the time he needs to do what he's been doing for many years, and in whose hands I feel safe and secure. When he says, 'Your lungs are perfect', and 'Your blood pressure and the oxygen levels in your blood are perfect', I am grateful to him and to my perfect body, even though it looks less … oh so much less! … than perfect.

What would it be like to have this man as your father?

I spent a third (or a quarter, if I'm lucky) of my life being disrespectful and ungrateful in art schools—the first ten years as a student, and then fifteen as a teacher—and for five of those years I was doing a doctorate in fine arts. It was the best possible education anyone could have, but the quality of an education depends more on the student and their mindset than on the teachers and the institution.

What would it be like to respect your father?

For centuries, they told the peasants in my grandmother's village that they had to be grateful to their lord and masters. And they were. And so we, who are now in the prime of our lives, or just past it, we too used to be told to respect our elders, our parents, the priest, the people with money—but we didn't like being told that, and so we didn't. But we had no ethics. Our ethics consisted of *Fuck You!*, and *We'll do as we fucking-well please. And don't try and stop us. And get off your high horse.* We were full of hate and loathing. And it felt good.

But what every human being really needs to learn are two things that are increasingly rare in educational institutions, but which you can find in any hospital by the bucketful—namely, gratitude and respect. And for this human being, during this year of working in a cancer hospital, learning how to engage with human beings who are dying, or who are afraid that they are going to die, you learn to be grateful. Or rather, it's not so much that you *learn* to be grateful; it's more a case of finding gratitude—and respect—arising within you.

And now you are walking outside, effortlessly filling your lungs with air, and moving your legs boldly, energetically forward, and singing, 'I've got two legs from my arse to the ground and ...'

This is to the tune of *The Lumberjack Song*, and this is when you find yourself swelling with gratitude, not directed *at* anyone or even *for* anything in particular. It's just being here and now ... free and unencumbered, and you're doing something that is meaningful and, to some extent, useful—and you're doing it with the entirety of your being. And you're doing it with respect.

Because gratitude begets respect, which is equally rare and just as important in this work.

Angelo says

Angelo says, 'You lucky!'

He is immobile, waiting, hoping ... to regain the use of his legs.

'I know.'

i know angelo i know how lucky i am i do now now now and

now and i am grateful and now and now and now each breath each step each moment yes yes yes …

Angelo said the doctor told him, 'We've all got to go some time …'

His luck ran out. And your luck can run out any time. Angelo told me this.

'That's life, mate …!'

Today, you are grateful to be alive, to be able to use your legs to negotiate space and gravity and your memory to negotiate time.

Today you're grateful to Angelo, for the reminder.

The new stoma

In room 5 is Ron, who is fifty-nine. Gravity has not been kind to him.

Oh my God, is that me in five year's time?

Ron regrets having 'the procedure' done. I'm waiting for him to tell me more when a nurse comes in. 'When did you last open your bowels, Ron?' he asks.

'A week ago last Friday,' Ron says, wistfully.

He had the procedure done on Monday. But what the nurse wants to know is whether his new stoma is active. It's just an awkward way of putting it. Ron doesn't know, and he doesn't want to know.

'I wish I hadn't told anyone,' he says to me.

'About …'

'My cancer.'

I nod.

'The mistake I made, you know the mistake I made?'

I shake my head.

'I told my sister! We've always been close. And she says, "You're having treatment!"'

He raises his eyebrows and makes his eyes big, I am guessing in a parody of his sister's face when she was telling him.

Ron has been incapable of carrying out his trade, which is welding. He tells me he's been redeployed as a kind of storeman, packing and unpacking things that need to be welded or that have been welded. And now he's just a few months away from retiring. He only has enough money to last him maybe five or six years.

'And then what?'

There is a tear or two. He says, 'Oh well' a lot, and 'We'll have to see.' He'll go back to Templestowe with his stoma, and he'll either get used to it or not. And he'll either go back to welding for a few months — or not. Probably not.

After a while, he says, 'You must have other people to see.'

'Yes, I do.'

'Well, I don't want to be holding you up …'

'Are you telling me to piss off?' I ask with a smile.

'If I knew you better, I probably would have told you to piss off.'

So I do. And Ron will be gone tomorrow, or not. And he will come back, or not. And I might see him again, or not — probably not. Such is the nature of this work.

Eduardo

Barbara has arranged a family meeting for Eduardo, who is seventy-eight years old. He's been in the hospital for a long time, and he's sick of being there. I haven't had much to do with him. His English is not great. All I've managed to get out of him is that he's from Sicily and that he used to be a soccer player. He has managed to communicate his extreme boredom and his unhappiness about being confined to a hospital and being poked and prodded all day.

His wife is in a nursing home 'with mental-health issues', but he has two supportive sons who visit often, usually wearing immaculate suits. Barbara says it would be good if I was able to be at the family meeting to support him, since he's going to be told that his prognosis is poor. I said I'd be glad to, but only if he wants me there. She suggests I speak with him and his family to find out if they would like me to attend the meeting. And so I do. Eduardo is not enthusiastic.

'We are not so far yet …!'

I take this to mean that he is not about to die and that a pastor, which is what he thinks I am, is not required yet. I explain that I can just be a calm, supportive presence in the room, and that may be helpful. When the sons say they think it's a good idea, their father readily agrees. He seems overwhelmed. He tells me he is 'cranky!'

The meeting goes for well over an hour. The surgeon explains that there are few options remaining for treatment due to the infection that has been caused by the progress of the disease. He proposes more antibiotics and more tests, but he says they must now 'begin to consider other options'. Some of these options are outlined by Barbara—hospice, high-needs care facility—and a few questions are asked of her by the sons. There is an uncomfortable silence that goes on for several minutes. Eduardo himself has said nothing. He's not making eye contact with anyone, and he looks shell-shocked.

I hear myself saying, 'What is it that *you* would like, Eduardo? Where would you like to be when there are no more options for treatment?'

Everyone is relieved. Eduardo says he wants to be somewhere where he can have his own room, and a TV with Foxtel for his sport. And he wants to be nearer to where his sons live, so they don't have to travel as far to visit him after a long day at work.

'That's all,' he says simply.

And the next day I am grateful for Eduardo's gratitude. I drop in on him to see how he is after yesterday. I'm a bit worried because he has somehow managed to interpret what the doctor said as a cause for optimism. And it's the first time I think I've heard the D-word being uttered by Eduardo.

'I thought I was going to die in here ...'

He looks at me for confirmation. I'm not sure I've heard him properly. He speaks with a thick accent.

'I beg your pardon?'

You don't want to be thinking you heard the D word if you didn't. Then he says it again.

How wrong can you be? I can hear him thinking. I am worried that he *will* die in here.

'So you don't want to die in the hospital?'

'No! It's terrible in here! Terrible! Let me go to another hospital closer to Geelong, so it's easier for my family to visit.

Or to a nice hops … hosp … what you call it?'

'Hospice?'

'Exactly. With Foxtel. So I can see the football.'

I don't know if there are any hospices with Foxtel; but if there are, his sons look like they could afford it. I just hope they're not tight-arses.

Apart from that, the only other problem is Eduardo's fever. It's a matter of getting that under control. Or finding out what is causing it, and getting that under control. Something is not right somewhere, but they don't know what it is. And you can't discharge someone with fever to a hospice. They wouldn't take him. Ironically, you have to be relatively well to get into to a hospice — especially, I suspect, one with Foxtel. The only thing that's allowed to be wrong with you when you go into a hospice is that you are dying.

Eduardo tells me how grateful he was for my presence at the meeting.

'You're the only one who's asked me what I want since I've been in this bloody place!'

I am silent.

'I want you at every meeting now.'

'That might not be possible, but I'll try!'

'Thank you … thank you …'

The old man pulls the sheet up around the top of his legs, and covers his penis and scrotum. They have been staring at me during the entire conversation.

'And I thank you, Eduardo.'

Barbara smiles at me as I'm getting into the lift and she's coming out.

'Thanks for yesterday, Johannes. It was really useful to have you there.'

'Pleasure. Thanks for inviting me. He says he wants me at every meeting now.'

'OK ...'

'But I'll be gone by the end of next month. My internship is almost finished.'

'Pity.'

'It is. But as long as I am here ...'

'OK. See you then.'

'See you, Barbara!'

The enema

'Hello! I'm Johannes from Pastoral Care.'

'I'm just about to have an enema.'

'OK. I can come back later, if you like.'

'Oh no.'

'What about tomorrow then?'

'Oh, well, I'm terminally ill now, so I've come to my own conclusions.'

'Well, sometimes it's helpful to talk to someone.'

'Oh no.'

'Not at all?'

'No.'

'No worries at all then. All the best.'

'Bye bye.'

Strange days indeed

These are strange days. But it's difficult to put your finger on exactly what it is that's strange. It's not just that these are my last weeks as a pastoral-care intern. It is as if there are small details that are just ever so slightly ... different. The hospital is almost eerily quiet. There are no referrals in the handover report, and I contemplate just sitting there and reading my book, and not going to the ward at all.

But then, of course, you go—not because you *have* to go. You could easily not go; if you're really needed, they will call you. But you go because you ought to go. And because you want to go. And because, even though you're not getting paid, it's your job. And if you don't go, no one will be there.

The ward seems deserted, except for Henri in the handover room. She is carefully spreading very thin layers of Vegemite on tiny biscuits.

'Hello! It's very quiet around here ...' I say cheerfully.

I learned early on that no matter how quiet it is on a ward, most people who work in the hospital avoid remarking on it for fear of being perceived as the cause when it suddenly becomes not quiet, but the words are out of my mouth before I realise.

Henri looks up and smiles.

'Ssssssh!'

She's been on all night and, for whatever reason—maybe someone called in sick—she's doing a double shift. Perhaps she's entered that peculiar space where the brain chemistry is altered through lack of sleep and it affects you like a contact high. There is absolutely no one around, and not a single sound can be heard. Maybe the apocalypse has come, and Henri and I are the only people in the world left alive.

'What's it like out there?' Henri says, and puts a biscuit in her mouth.

People don't usually talk about 'out there' when they're 'in here'. In all the time I have spent in the hospital, and in all the conversations I have had with nurses, I can count on the fingers of one hand the number of times someone who works there has talked to me about the world beyond the hospital.

'Sunny. Quite cold, but beautiful,' I say. 'You should get out there. Have a break.'

'The patient in 9 is still hanging on. She is on day 4 of the Liverpool Care Plan,' Henri says, swallowing.

'I'll go and have a look.'

The person in 9 is unconscious, but seems comfortable. The tired-looking son is in the room with her. He's been there all night. He has a laptop open on the table in front of him.

'Trying to write an essay for uni,' he says apologetically.

Life goes on.

'Can't you get an extension? In view of the circumstances?'

His mother groans a little.

'I don't want one! It'll just cut into the time I need to work on the next one that's due!'

The university seems a long, long way away.

'What's it on?'

'Lacan.'

'Really? Interesting!'

We discuss Lacan, and his relevance or otherwise. It seems a little odd to be discussing psychoanalysis with someone whose mother is in the room, dying, in a deserted hospital, but it's no odder than lots of other things I have experienced this year. And he seems to have forgiven her. I was reading an interview with a Lacanian psychoanalyst who says that in the Lacanian way of working, the analyst, too, functions in a way similar to a clown.

Edna

'Hey, Em! How are you?' I say to the nurse in charge as I walk into the ward.

'Good thanks. You?' Emma says brightly.

'Very good thanks … Any urgent referrals?'

'Not really … well …' she hesitates. 'Edna … but only if you've got time. It's not really urgent.'

'OK. I've got time. What's up?'

'She's pissed off.' Emma makes a face.

'My specialty,' I say with a grin. 'I'll go and see her now.'

'Thanks, Johannes.'

'No worries!'

It's not my ward, but I know the name. She has a reputation. I've heard she's been rude and difficult with staff and other pastoral workers.

I tell Edna who I am, and then I say, 'How are you going?'

'So-so.'

She is a large woman, but in all other respects she reminds me of someone else—same age, same disease, in the same place. Prognosis: negative.

'You've had enough?'

'Of what?'

'Being in here.'

'Yes.'

'Are you sad?'

'Of course!'

'Angry?'

'No.'

It's difficult for Edna to breathe, so it's not easy for her to talk, but she hasn't told me to go away. I decide not to wait for an invitation, and I sit down.

'What do you want me to say?' Edna says.

I'm looking at her and I am formulating an answer, but before I've a chance to say anything, she says, 'I'm not gonna make your job easy for you …!'

I smile.

'You don't have to make my job easy, Edna.'

Later, when I recall her saying this, even now as I'm writing this, it makes tears come. I wonder why …

She seems to relax a bit after she's asked what denomination I am and I've told her. She says she's not interested in thinking about death.

'That's OK. You don't have to think about it if you don't want to.'

She turned fifty the other day.

'Didn't ever think I'd get to that.'

I wait for her to say more.

'But that's life. That's how it goes. And you gotta be positive,' she says resignedly.

And that is how she's got through the ten years since she was first diagnosed with breast cancer. But now it's in her lungs, and she's finding it more and more difficult to breathe. We end up talking about it anyway. She thinks she's got maybe a few weeks.

'Who knows? Me lungs are fillin' up with fluid so fast—they drained two-and-a-half litres out a few days ago, and they're fillin' up again.'

Edna changes the subject. 'Why do you do this work?'

'To meet people like you!'

She snorts scornfully and asks how I lost my religion. I tell her the story.

'But,' I say, 'even though I don't believe in a god, I don't believe it's all meaningless. I believe in something. I just don't know what to call it, or how to understand it.'

Edna tells me she lost her dad when she was seventeen, and says she still talks to him. She describes how all her relatives on her father's side are on the kerb waiting to cross the road. Her father is already on the other side.

'But I think I'm gonna to be the first one to cross.' She weeps.

I almost say, *You'll be with him.* But I don't. It's too easy. And she won't. Not in the way that she wants to be, anyway.

'I think that's all I have to say, love,' Edna says.

I take her hand.

'That's OK.'

She grips my hand energetically.

'You have to trust, don't you?' I say.

She nods. A tear is rolling down her cheek.

'It doesn't matter that you don't know what to trust *in*. Trust in meaning, in order, in beauty. When you look at the stars, what do you see?'

The tear glistens.

And that's what I leave her with. That's all I've got. I've just given it to her.

She gives me a tired smile. I get up, say goodbye, and walk away. I take the stairs down to Intensive Care. I walk slowly. I have to think.

This is the point, isn't it? If you're an atheist in a foxhole and you want someone to come, you want someone to be there, you want that someone to be a non-believer. This is why I am here.

Harry is with Meg in Intensive Care. At first I think there is a different patient in the bed, but no, that's Harry standing there. And so that must be Meg he's talking to! He is showing her photographs and cards from all the well-wishers that have arrived while she was unconscious, which was for the best part of a fortnight. Everyone had secretly given up on her, except Harry. And there she is talking to him. They have taken the tubes out. I can't understand a single word she's saying, but I say, 'Wow! I haven't heard you talk before.'

They are both beaming.

And then I say, pointing at Harry, 'You can start telling him off now!'

'She already has,' Harry says drily.

Duty pastoral-carer report:

> Edna is tired of being in hospital and anxious. I provided
> a supportive listening environment. She is nearing end of

life. She is an atheist. We discussed what you *can* believe in when you are an atheist and we held hands.

Like I said, she reminds me of another person in the hospital who was also referred to pastoral care and described as difficult. She's dead now.

I miss her.

On knowing

I had two interactions with Fred during his previous admission. We chatted about computers — that's how we got talking initially. I'd been to see Ernie in the bed opposite, and I couldn't help but notice in passing that, on his little table, Fred had a Macbook Air, an iPad, and an iPhone. My relationship with Ernie was quite jocular, and I suppose that's why I said jokingly, 'Where's your iPod?'

He looked at me as if I'd just put a steaming, fresh turd on his immaculate backlit keyboard.

I said, by way of explanation, 'You've almost got a full suite of Apple products there!'

Without a hint of a smile, he said, 'It's in my bag.'

Sometimes, on the ward, you feel a bit like you've been caught looking through the window into someone's lounge room. To cover my discomfort, I told him I'd been using Apple computers since 1988. He said he was a recent convert. We had a chat about what great products they are, but I didn't get the feeling that he was keen on talking with me.

A day or two later, I was talking to Ernie in the bed opposite about football. He's a Carlton fan, and the conversation turned to the Tigers, and he said, 'You should talk to Fred over there. He goes for the Tigers!'

Fred wasn't in his bed, but when I saw him the next day I said, 'Ernie tells me you're a Tigers fan!'

He replied enthusiastically. I asked him what he thought of our chances of making the eight, and we chatted for a good twenty minutes. It was clear that here was a man who took football seriously. We had an in-depth conversation about several of our players and their merits or otherwise, and he impressed me with his knowledge and understanding of the game.

Fred expressed the hope that he would be well enough to go and see the Tigers play another game before the end of the season, which was a few weeks away, but then he began to wonder whether he would live long enough to see them win another flag. He became a little sad, but it was friendly and cordial, and I grew optimistic of one day having a deep and meaningful conversation with Fred. But by the next day, he had disappeared, as so often happens.

In the week after the grand final, Fred was readmitted. He spent a day on someone else's ward, had a medical emergency when I was off duty, and was moved into Intensive Care.

That morning I decide to sit in the sunshine for a few minutes on a park bench on the way to the hospital. I see a woman coming towards me. Her gait is a little odd. Our eyes meet, and she starts talking to me about herself at great length, and I provide a listening presence, as it's called in pastoral-care speak.

'I have a disability,' she says simply.

She tells me all about her life—the words tumbling out, falling over each other—and she asks me a few questions about mine, which I answer in the most minimal way possible. After a while, I start to feel like she will talk forever.

How do you know when you've said enough? When is it time to go? That is *knowing*. We've been talking about this in supervision. *How* do you know? You just know, don't you? But not if you have a dysfunctional brain, or if you are on medication that interferes with its functioning so that you miss all kinds of subtle cultural cues and conventions.

She doesn't leave a lot of gaps in the stream of words, so in the end I just stand up and say, 'I've got to go! See you later.' And I am gone.

By this stage, I am the pastoral worker for the Intensive Care Unit, and I say hello to Fred and ask how he is going.

'I've turned a corner! I am going back to the ward today.'

'Well, that must be good!'

We make some small talk about the Tigers' last game of the season, which has ended in a draw—something that rarely happens in Australian Rules Football—and how we didn't make the finals again. I really don't think it is going to be more than a five-minute conversation, and I am conscious of having other patients to see. But by now I often feel that I am able to pick up when someone needs to talk. It's not really a skill, as such—it's mostly intuitive—but the intuitive function is augmented by experience. And that's what I mean by *knowing*.

Fred tells me he's looking forward to having a shower. He's wearing a *Metallica* T-shirt, and I make a joke about that—something about how you're *supposed* to be smelly if you're wearing a *Metallica* T-shirt. He tells me his wife has gone to Bali with her best friend for a holiday.

'When I was admitted she wanted to cancel it, but I persuaded her to go.'

'Yeah ... that's difficult, isn't it? You don't want to be the cause of someone cancelling their holiday, especially when there is nothing they can actually do.'

'Exactly. And they'd been planning this trip for a long time.'

'But it's understandable that, for them, it's difficult to have a good time when they're worrying about you.'

'The main thing is, I'm worried about what my family will think when they hear she has gone.'

'Oh?'

And then I think I hear him say something about being worried about his father. It is almost inaudible, as though his voice has cracked, but I'm not sure if this is just an effect of his illness. Then he says something else about going back to the ward—I can't quite pick it up—and then there is a pause.

He is looking down at his hands and arms, which are covered in some sort of red dye. And then I say it.

'Did I hear you say something about being worried about your father?'

'Yes.' He pauses. 'I'm upset about my father. They gave him the last rites two weeks ago, but he's still hanging on. And now I'm in here.'

'Oh, I am sorry.' I reach out and put my hand on his forearm. 'Are you close to your father?'

'Yes. Very much so,' he says. He lets out one, two, big loud sobs.

He recovers himself quickly and tells me he married 'late.' He is sad about having spent less time with his father since he was married. But they've had some good conversations in recent times, as it's become clear that his father doesn't have long to live. Fred says he feels 'everything's been sorted out' between them.

He sobs again. 'I'm sorry. I don't usually do this.'

'Don't be sorry!'

He is trying to talk through the tears, but then he gives up. He keeps getting angry with himself when he cries. Every time he starts crying, he says, 'Fred!' in an exasperated way.

'It's OK.'

We sit together in silence for quite a while. All around us, the critical-care unit is on full swing. People are having procedures done. Machines beep and bleep. Medical staff are going to and fro. We don't even have the curtain closed around us. We are an island.

'I've never spoken with anybody about this. I do feel a lot better. Thank you so much for listening to me,' he says.

'No worries. Any time.'

His nurse comes over when I am talking to Eve about another patient in the handover room.

'What's happening with Fred?' she asks.

She's concerned about him, and hasn't been able to find out what is bothering him.

'Yeah,' I say, in a non-committal way. 'He's working through some personal stuff.'

The next day, Fred has been moved to my ward. At the ward meeting, the nurse unit-manager says, 'I don't know what's going on with this man. He seems anxious, but he's a very closed, private person. Maybe you should see him,' she says to Elizabeth, the psychologist.

I mention that I spent an hour with Fred in the ICU yesterday.

'Can I see you about this patient after the meeting?' Elizabeth says.

Elizabeth asks a lot of questions, and it's not as easy to deflect them as those of the nurse or the woman in the park. I'm uncomfortable, but I'm conscious of the fact that I'm a member of a team in an institution that is responsible for looking after Fred. I feel obliged to answer her questions, but that's all I do. I can protect the confidences he shared with me by not volunteering any information. I guess I am making a contribution to the knowledge the institution has about him in the hope that it will benefit him. I'm aware that there is also an economy of knowledge at work here. The hospital *wants* to know — because it values knowledge — and people want to know details because they *like* knowing.

And what of the knowing? Who really knows the patient? Who is engaged with the patient in a process of knowing? I feel as though I betrayed Fred. And now, writing it, writing a book? If he reads this, he may well recognise himself, but no one else would. I have left out most of what Fred told me, using only the bare bones of what I needed to tell the story, and changing the most crucial details.

Knowledge is a burden, but knowing isn't.

Are we there yet?

One of the things that is required of pastoral-care interns is that every three months they present a document about their 'spiritual journey'. I don't like 'journey' as a metaphor for development or change. It makes me think of sitting on a train with the landscape unfolding around me. Much as I like trains and travel, I usually have a big bag of stuff with me, the train is running late, and I've had to stand around on a draughty platform waiting for it. For me, change and development is not linear and progressive like a journey on a train or, for that matter, by car or bicycle or on foot. 'Becoming' happens haphazardly in a number of different directions all at once—or not at all—then quickly and slowly, and then imperceptibly. You're not in one place on your way to another. You're just here, that's all. And then you're not.

How can we say what we are *now*? And now? And now? And are we there yet? And what if, when we get there, 'There is no there there,' as Gertrude Stein observed about the city of Oakland.

Some people talk in terms of a 'cancer journey'. I also avoid the word 'journey' when I'm talking to people in the hospital about their experience of the disease. There is change, of course, and there are changing contexts, and the way we make meaning depends on the context. There are changing meanings and relationships. Music changes as we listen; it is changed by the act of listening. And likewise what we see changes, too, and how we interpret what we see. I am a different man today from the man I was yesterday. I've changed. Each day the question is asked. Some days, we have the energy to answer it.

Some days, we have the courage to let it hang in the air. Some days, we are at great pains to move around it.

So, life is an artwork, and the artist is sometimes a priest and sometimes a clown. And so is the pastoral worker. The key is knowing *when* to be a priest and *when* to be a clown. For years, my view of art was like David Foster Wallace's idea about literature being like giving CPR to those elements of what is human and magical that are still alive in these dark times, and to illuminate the possibilities of being human.

And then I could find no way to continue making art, so I stopped. And Wallace could find no way to continue, and thus he failed, too. What a waste. But yes. *To illuminate the possibilities for being alive and human in the world.* I tried and failed to do that by making and teaching art and writing about it. That was thirty years of my life I'll never get back. But now? Maybe I've found a way—a humble, minimalist way. And maybe there is a way that this book can become art.

Jazz for Jacob

There is loud jazz music coming out of the room in which a man called Jacob is not busy being born. There is only one thing left for him to do in his life, and that is to die. But today—here, now—he is still breathing. And then he stops. It is quiet—but his body is trembling, shuddering almost. Is that his heart beating? It would otherwise be eerily quiet; maybe that's why the nurse turned on the jazz. I am thinking about whether Jacob likes jazz, and whether I would like it if loud jazz was playing as I lay dying. And then the laboured, irregular breathing starts up again.

'I spoke to him loudly,' my colleague said yesterday, 'but he did not respond.' That's exactly how he said it, in that formal way. Today, I don't say anything to Jacob. I walk in quietly and turn off the jazz. Then I put my hand on his bruised and weather-beaten arm. It is stone cold, but he is still breathing.

I go back in the afternoon. The nurse told me he never has any visitors. The jazz has been turned on again, but it's not as loud as before. Jacob is still breathing on and off, and one of his eyes is half-open. I go and stand in front of the half-open eye, and there it is, my compassion. It's strange: since I've come back to work after a weekend off, I haven't felt the same connection with it.

I want to say, *There, there, old man. It's time to go. It's all right. You can let go now.*

But I don't say it; I only think it. Maybe that's enough.

If he's still alive tomorrow morning, I will go and tell him.

Sometimes it seems like the hospital is an organism, and that sometimes it catches a fever. When I leave the hospital, two men are dying on my ward; when I come back the next day, one is dead and the other one isn't. Jacob died around six o'clock. The other man has a son and an estranged daughter. Both were called. He came; she didn't. I am standing in the room with the dying man and his son.

'It won't be long now,' I say softly. *But that's what I thought yesterday. How long is not long?* 'It's possible that he can still hear you, but he's unable to respond. If there is something you want to say to him, you should say it.'

'It's as if he's hanging on,' the son mutters.

'Is there any chance of your sister …?'

'Yes. She's on her way.'

I feel like asking why she hasn't spoken to him for so long, but this is not the time, and it's none of my business. None of this is any of my business, really, but where they lead, I follow. That's what my business is. And the dying. That is my core business.

The stupidity of people

My dreams are full of highly competent young women with cool heads and sensible hair whom you would trust with your life. But this afternoon they are all crowded around Richard, who is suddenly experiencing problems with his heart. Luckily, he's got Lucy, his partner. She is a gem.

'If he can see that I am here, he'll be all right,' Lucy says. And he is.

Talking to John, my stepfather, on the phone last night about something or other, the conversation ended up, as it often does, with him expressing incredulity about the stupidity of people.

But John, I wanted to say, *everyday I meet people who are incredibly intelligent and courageous and generous. Maybe you're not hanging out in the right places. Or maybe you watch too much TV. That's also possible. There are a lot of stupid people on TV.*

But I didn't say that. I said, 'Yes, John.'

The Buddha nature of Bob's uncle

Gerald tells me today that he wouldn't have made it without me. Someone else said that to me once, too. That seems like a long time ago.

His penultimate round of chemo is finished, but they kept him in for a couple of days and gave him a course of IV antibiotics because he had a fever. Today he is all clear and is being discharged. I call in to say goodbye. I tell him that my internship is almost over and I won't be here when he comes in for his final round of chemo.

'I wanted to thank you for all you've done to support me,' Gerald says. He pronounces each word carefully, as if he's been rehearsing a speech.

'It's been an absolute pleasure, Gerald.'

He reminds me of the time when he was very low and I gave him my hand. 'I don't know if you remember …'

I remember. We'd had a lengthy session. I remember how he gripped my hand, and I answered him by gripping back. We stayed like that for quite a while.

Gerald says that gave him strength, and enabled him to pull himself together. 'I could feel the *power* coming from you!' he says, and looks at me intently. It is as if I enter a dimension where all time is contained in the present and, sitting there in the half dark with the glowing Gerald, his keen eyes watching me, I remember.

I am standing at the door; I was just passing by, and I wanted to see how Gerald was going. But with Gerald, as with other patients on the ward who are in isolation, I first like to make sure they are willing and able to see me, because you don't want to go to the trouble of gowning up and putting on gloves if they are tired and/or they don't feel like talking. It is always awkward gowning up. It doesn't take me as long as it used to, and it doesn't take me as long as the old priest who visits the Catholics in the hospital on Wednesdays—but he is in his late seventies. Sometimes when I see him struggling, I stop to help him get into his gown, or to pull the gloves down over his arthritic fingers.

'Hi, Gerald. How are you?'

He motions for me to come in.

'I've been hoping you would come by. Come in. Come in … if you've got time. I want to tell you something.'

He seems a bit hyper. 'Hang on. I'll just gown up.'

Gerald is always respectful of my time. I've told him to ask the nurse to page me if he needs to talk, but I don't think he would ever do that. It's just not his thing; he wouldn't want to impose himself. When I walk into the room, Gerald is glowing. He says his lymphoma has completely disappeared from his abdomen. The doctor came and told him the results of the latest scans today.

'Wow. That is amazing!'

I don't say, *I told you so!*

I never say, *I told you so.* People either remember that you told them so, or they don't. And sometimes they don't want to remember. They want to feel like they thought of it themselves first. And what does it matter that you told them so? My mother is always telling me that she told me so, even when she didn't. But Gerald remembers.

This was on Friday. Gerald was happy. This was before Bob's mother came in and told him Bob was dead.

I remember when Bob died.

I receive a message on my pager saying Bob has died, late on Friday afternoon. I've been thinking about how soon after five I can get out of the hospital. It has been a long week and, like all the other workers in the hospital who are not on duty until Monday, I am keen to get home to have my dinner and begin the relaxing weekend I have planned.

Earlier today, the nurse in charge told me that Bob was 'not for pastoral care,' so I didn't go in and see him. But when I arrive on the ward, the social worker asks me to arrange for a Greek Orthodox priest to come and do whatever it is that they do when someone dies.

'Orthodox people usually prefer to have their own local priest come,' I say. 'Is that what they want?' The social worker doesn't know. The next minute, I am in the room with a dead man and his grieving family.

Bob's eyes are half open, and this might seem like an obvious observation, but I am always struck by how *lifeless* a dead person is. It might just be because I *know* that they are dead, and that they will never move any part of themselves again. They are no longer *able to Be*, as Heidegger puts it.

I offer my condolences, and tell them there is a number I can call to get a Greek Orthodox priest to come, and they are happy with that. Several more family members come into the room. They've only just been told that Bob is dead, but they haven't seen him yet, and when they do, they begin sobbing loudly. I am in two minds as to whether to stay with the family and console them, or to go and do my priest-finding duty. I stand there with them for a while. They are completely focused on the dead man, staring at him as though they can't believe it, and perhaps they can't yet. Seeing the dead person can be an important part of processing the fact that he or she is no longer alive.

I decide the best thing I can do for this family is to go and make arrangements for a priest to come. They are all supporting each other.

I ring about half-a-dozen numbers before I get any response at all, and then it is as if the priest is reluctant to come. He wants to talk to the family. I feel like saying, *What is your problem? Someone has died. Can you just come over and do your job already?*

The height of absurdity is reached when the priest hangs up on me. I had been having trouble understanding him, and I had to keep asking him to repeat what he had just said. Eventually, I do manage to find a priest who is reasonable. He asks me to give him the direct number of the ward, and says he will ring and talk to the family.

I go back to the ward to let them know, and when the lift doors open, Bob's wife, Zelda, is standing right there, talking intently with another family member. I stop to tell her I am sorry. To my great surprise, she puts out her arms for a hug, and then, as we are standing there with our arms around each other, I am there *with* them.

The other family member is saying many good things to Zelda. He's doing a fantastic job of pastoral care. Zelda is laughing and crying, and she keeps looking at me for confirmation. I am nodding, and smiling my weary, sad smile.

'This is how it is. This is how it has to be,' he keeps saying to Zelda. 'This is it. It's up to you now. You have to make a new life for yourself.'

And I am thinking, *He is right. This is it. And these are the moments that you do it for, this work. This is what makes it all meaningful. Today it is this, and the minutes I had with Charlie this morning sitting next to him, talking about Rose. And I said to him, 'Hang in there, mate. You'll get there.' He doesn't ask me where 'there' is, and he doesn't say the thing Gertrude Stein said about Oakland.*

And today it's Gerald, and Bob's uncle, whose name I don't even know. And tomorrow it will be someone else. Later, I am standing outside with Bob's uncle. He is coughing and smoking a cigarette, and he is sad but philosophical.

'He works hard,' Bob's uncle is saying. 'Seven days a week. He never swears. Every night I pray. But in the end I said, "You want him. You take him." That's it.'

And then I am thinking, *Yes, he's right. That's it. Bob is dead. These people are all fucking Buddhas. What am I even doing here?*

Radar Love

I remember how much Gerald was affected by Bob's death. I can't remember who referred him—maybe no one. I am my own referral. I find my own rhythm. I listen. I make mental notes. No, I am sure someone said, 'Gerald is upset about Bob.' Maybe it was the patient in the next room, Maureen. For some reason, Bob's mother went into Maureen and Gerald's rooms and told them that Bob was dead. This doesn't usually happen in the hospital, but maybe she just needed to tell someone.

Maureen and Gerald are about the same age as Bob, and they're both upset, even though neither really knew him.

To Maureen, I say, 'Well, Maureen, you just have to keep your hands on the wheel and your eyes on the road. Don't you?'

I always think that's from 'Radar Love', but it's not. It's from 'Roadhouse Blues' by The Doors. I don't know if she gets the reference or not, but Maureen agrees: 'Yes ... Otherwise you end up wrapped around a tree by the side of the road.'

'Exactly. So let's remember Bob and pay our respects to his family, and then focus on getting well.'

They both want to get well. So then I go and see Gerald. I tell him the same thing. I don't know if either of them have ever heard the song—they might be too young—but it is playing over and over in my head right now. Gerald says he's sorry he never went in to say hello to Bob. He talked to the wife and the mother in the day room, but he only stood at the door and waved to Bob.

'But Gerald, you wouldn't have been allowed in. Bob was in isolation. His immune system was shot to pieces. You were highly infectious. You could have killed him,' I say.

'That's true. I wouldn't have been allowed in, would I?'

I walk around the side of the bed where Gerald is sitting so I can look him in the eyes. He always has the blinds drawn and the lights off.

'No!' I say. I can barely see his eyes. 'You're a good man, Gerald.'

I take his hand. He grips it hard. We did this another time, months ago, when he was in the middle of his first chemo. He was quiet then. He just looked at me, and I just stood there.

And now this

I am remembering the first time I met Gerald. He told me that his wife had died, of breast cancer. She was the love of his life. He has a son from that marriage. He is in his late twenties now.

'How is your relationship with him?'

'Good. Good! Now … '

'It wasn't before?'

He hesitates. 'Oh, well. On and off, you know. His mother died of cancer, and now I've got this.'

'But it's good now?'

'Yes. He visits me. He keeps me sane. I can discuss things with him, you know.'

He got married again. He had another son, but the marriage broke down. 'She took me to the cleaners,' Gerald says sadly. He lost everything—his house, his business, his son. *And now this.*

He misses him terribly.

'And how old is your other son?'

'Four. He is four years old now. I love him so much. '

'And do you get to see him?'

'Yes. I get to see him. Once a fortnight.'

'You're amazing! How do you keep going? How do you keep your spirits up?'

He looks up at the ceiling.

'Him. Up there. He looks after me.'

His faith is important to him. He prays every night.

'Better must come, hey, Gerald?'

'You think so?'

'Yes. Believe it. You deserve it.'

None of this is textbook pastoral care, but it doesn't matter anymore. I've passed my advanced certificate. I'm post-advanced now — whatever that means. And now Gerald is saying, 'I wouldn't have made it without you.'

The textbook response to this would be, 'Ah, Gerald it wasn't me. It was you. You did it yourself. It was your strength that got you through — not mine.'

But this was his experience; he needed someone to be there. And I was *good enough*. His experience was that I was there for him. My job is to enable him to find his own strength, but for now he feels like he is able to use mine, and it's OK.

It is not that you need these moments, or expect them — or even hope for them — to make this work worthwhile, but it makes a huge difference. You see, you want to do something. Something that changes things, even if only slightly, for people who are suffering. That's why you came to his place. That's why you chose to do this work rather than the other work.

In any case, this is why we are all here. Or it should be. That's why we, who are not sick, come to this place. And that's why I am grateful to Gerald today. Because he took the time to name what he experienced as my gift to him, and to thank me for it. That's why I left the other place. Because the only difference my being there was making was to my bank balance. Not to people. Not really. Maybe sometimes, rarely, a little. But not like this.

I give him my card.

'I will always remember you,' he says.

I thank him.

'And me you,' I tell him, and we shake hands for the last time. We grip hard.

Lillian

I only encounter one person who refuses pastoral care from me because I am a non-believer. I've previously had an amicable-enough encounter with Lillian when she was on another ward. Patients get moved around. They often go into the Intensive Care Unit for at least 24 hours after major surgery before they are moved on to the ward, or there may not be a bed available on the ward where the patient should go, and they are temporarily given a bed on another ward and moved when a bed becomes available.

The colleague who has previously worked with Lillian on the other ward rolls her eyes when she mentions her to me at handover. 'Lillian wants to become a nun,' she says, 'but they won't have her because of her cancer.'

A sheet is tightly drawn around up to her neck, from which protrudes a large, hairless head with big, brown eyes looking around anxiously. Lillian seems permanently startled. The head and eyes appear bigger when someone has no hair, and Lillian has no eyebrows either, due to the chemo. She has a broad Australian accent and a kind of nasal twang, like Kath, or Kim—I can never remember which is which—and she says 'and that' a lot. She tells me about her brother John, who was so good to her when she was growing up, always looked after her at school 'and that', and now he's in another hospital with cancer, and she doesn't know if she will ever see him again.

'Can you talk to him on the phone?'

'Yeah, I can, but it's not the same,' she says dismissively. 'Anyway, it makes me too sad and that. I wouldn't know what to say.'

'You could tell him how much he ...'

'I just want to see him. To give him a hug and that.'

I don't remember how we got onto the topic, but Lillian asks me what I believe, and because I can't think of something lighter, I say something about the eleven dimensions and the ten-to-the-power-of-five-hundred universes, and the countless electrons and protons and fermions and quarks that multiply endlessly, even as we speak, and that appear and disappear as we are looking at them, but that can never occupy the same space or have the same velocity or momentum.

'A universe could be forming right here right now in this room, and we wouldn't even know it!'

She looks at me incredulously; the eyes appear even bigger.

'Anyway, that's what Sean Carroll says,' I add. 'He's a professor of physics.'

'But you don't believe in God the father?'

'No, I don't.'

It didn't seem to be an issue that day.

In my clinical report, I didn't mention the fermions and the quarks. I wrote:

> I discussed religious and spiritual needs with Lillian and
> we had a wide-ranging and agreeable conversation about
> our beliefs and the meaning of a good life. Lillian said she
> is Church of England. I offered to find her a Christian
> pastoral worker but she said she was happy to talk to me.
> I made her aware of the Sunday service which she said
> she would very much like to attend if she is able.

But that was then, and this is now. It is late on a Friday night. Outside, the city's workers' celebrations of the arrival of the weekend are in full swing, but Lillian is in a great deal of distress and I am the duty pastoral worker. Carla the unflappable, impeccable nurse in charge on Ward 5, who reminds me of Agent Olivia Dunham in *Fringe*, has called me in to the hospital.

'Lillian,' is the only thing Carla says when I get there.

Carla is not the kind of person who would roll their eyes when speaking of a patient to another staff member, like my colleague in the handover meeting, but if she was, she would have.

You can hear Lillian weeping and wailing from down the corridor. When she sees me, she starts crying even louder, and sobs, 'They told me a Christian lady pastoral worker would come.'

'Lillian, it's after hours. I am the only worker on duty now.'

She continues to weep. 'I really wanted a priest.'

'We have a priest coming in on Sunday to do the service.

Can you come to the service?'

She says she can't wait until Sunday. She is extremely agitated. A nurse I've never seen before arrives to check on her. Lillian complains of being hot, and then of being cold. When the nurse leaves, Lilian says, 'It is so dark. I'm afraid.'

She weeps bitterly.

'Tell me about your fear.'

'What's the point?' she cries out impatiently. 'You're not a Christian!'

I can think of nothing to say to that.

'I just want it all to be all over.'

'It's not time yet.'

She continues to weep.

'Give me your hand.'

She shakes her head. I say nothing. I am quite calm.

'I'll be back soon.'

I walk back to the office. Lady Gaga is in town, and there are all kinds of strange-looking, excited young people milling around outside. One of the nurses told me that Gaga is staying in the hotel next door. In the office, all the lights are off, as is the air conditioning. It's very stuffy, and I am finding it hard to breathe. It is 10.30 pm, but I will have to ring the consultant. The consultant, who is an off-duty senior worker, usually—but not always—the head of department, is available for consultation by telephone for the duty pastoral worker should the need arise.

'Gird your loins,' is the consultant's advice.

She sounds sleepy.

'Go back in. Be firm. You are the duty pastoral worker, and unless she is dying, no priest will want to come. That's it. If she refuses pastoral care from you, tell her someone can come in the morning, and go home.'

Lillian is a bit calmer when I get back. I have a whole speech ready, but I just say, 'Give me your hand,' again.

This time she takes her hand from underneath the blanket and puts it in mine. It is very hot.

What do you think God's plan for you is?'

'I don't know. I'm just so afraid and that,' she sobs.

'Can you pray?'

'Yes.'

'So you have to pray and put your trust in God. Don't you?'

'Yes, but I love Him so much. I just want to be with Him now.'

'But isn't he everywhere ?'

'Yes … ?'

'Well, then, he is with you now, and you are with him!'

'Yes.'

There is a pause. She is beginning to breathe more easily.

'It is just that sometimes He seems so far away.'

'I know.'

We sit together in silence for a while.

'Are you OK now?'

She nods.

'Try to get some sleep …'

'OK.'

I would never have thought it possible for a non-believer to console a Christian, but there it is. In a way, it is like speaking German. I don't really speak German, but Dutch is my mother tongue, so I know how to make noises that sound like German, and I know some German words. And when I don't know a word I just say the Dutch word with a German accent, and I wave my arms around. It seems to work. I get by.

A blessing

My encounter with Lillian was, in effect, a practical examination of the principle that a pastoral worker should be able to work with anyone, regardless of their faith or lack of faith. Of course, there are specific religious rituals that require an official from that tradition, but even a non-believer can do a blessing. I learned that from Jim, an old Catholic priest who was dying of cancer.

I'd had a good chat with Jim about the football and the weather. The only reason I knew he was a priest was because I had been told at handover. But when I was saying goodbye, he asked me for a blessing.

Shit! I hadn't bargained for that.

I had not outed myself to him as a non-believer. There seemed to be no need, and I didn't want to make a point of it, as it might have made him uncomfortable. But I guessed I had to now.

'I can't do that, Jim!'

'Why?!'

'I don't know how!'

'It's pretty bloody easy!' He seems incredulous.

'Maybe you can teach me?'

'OK,' he begins. 'Well, you have to think of God …'

'Well, that's a problem.'

'Why is that?'

'I don't believe in God!'

Even though I have considered myself a non-believer for more than forty years, I was brought up a Catholic, and to tell a priest you don't believe in God still makes the heart beat faster.

'Oh well ... I can't help you then,' Jim says sadly.

'What if I was to think about the universe, and everything that's good in it, and the good in people?' I said.

'OK,' Jim says. 'Try me!'

'Sorry?'

'Try me! Do what you're going to do, and I'll tell you if it worked.'

I put my hand on Jim's arm and I look into his sad, blue eyes for a few seconds. There is something of an old dog in them, one who has been frequently disappointed by his master. Then I take my hand away, and nod slightly.

'That's it?' Jim asks.

'That's it!'

'That will do me,' Jim says with a smile.

'You felt something? You felt a connection?'

'Certainly!'

'Thanks, Jim!'

'No, I thank you!'

There are numerous on-the-spot practical examinations in the life of a pastoral-care intern. And you usually know straight away whether you have passed or not.

Envoi

The story that forms the backbone of the book is my own story. And that story begins with another story, a ghost story told to me by my grandmother a long time ago. More than one hundred years ago, when my grandmother was a little girl, she saw the ghost of an old man standing by the foot of her bed. 'He was looking for something,' she said, 'he was always looking for something.'

She liked telling stories, my grandmother, but she had a limited repertoire. There were stories she could have told me that would have been worth telling, but she didn't—like how she became pregnant at the age of eighteen by the rich farmer for whom she worked as a servant. But she didn't want to tell me about that. These were things that were not talked about.

So she told me the same stories on more than one occasion, one of which was this one, and she described the ghost in great detail—the kind of pants he was wearing, rough sailor's pants. And one time he was in bare feet! And I believed her. It was the details that made me believe her.

My grandmother timed her death carefully. She chose to die as my plane was landing at Schiphol after what had been a seven-year absence from my motherland. I had been looking forward to seeing her, but also dreading it. She had become bitter in the old people's home. She was virtually immobile, nothing pleased her, and she hated the food there. She'd had enough. My mother was waiting at the airport, but I didn't even recognise her at first — she had grown so old and tired. We were at home having coffee when the phone rang. My mother was devastated by the news, and I was there to support her. My grandmother had made sure of that.

I believe that my grandmother believed she saw a ghost, but I am a non-believer. I don't believe in an afterlife, and I don't subscribe to the idea of spiritual beings or a spiritual realm. The idea of some kind of individual spiritual essence that continues to exist after the body dies, and which is somehow recognisable as the person that once was, seems such a solipsistic idea, so inwardly focused and imprecise — like bad science fiction.

'Spiritual' seems to be a word that people who wouldn't think of themselves as religious use when they mean 'something meaningful but immaterial, ineffable, unknowable'. Yet despite, or perhaps because of, the fact that everyone has a different idea of what 'spiritual' means, there is a growing tendency to call 'pastoral care', which has quite a precise meaning and a long history, 'spiritual care'.

OK, so there may be no such thing as an atheist in a foxhole, but there are those for whom resisting the urge for transcendence is a principle to which they are as deeply committed as any religious person is to the opposite. What kind of pastoral care do *they* need?

When you start defining something, it provides an opportunity for everyone to disagree with your definition, because everyone has their own understanding of what it is, and everyone is invested in *how* they understand it. Let's come to an understanding of what something is gradually, by telling our stories, by listening to others' stories, and sharing our experiences. And this is how we may come to understand what we have in common, as well as how we're different. This is how we could begin.

And perhaps what we have in common is that we are prepared to consider the questions that have been on the minds of human beings since they first had minds: *What does it mean to be a human being?* And from that flows the other question: *What does it mean to live?* And: *What does it mean to die?* And then we want to know: *What is a good life?* and *What is a good death?*

And we are prepared to engage in open dialogue about these questions, and this is what is important to people in the foxhole: that there are people who are prepared to listen and to talk with you about what it means to be here.

Acknowledgements

I would like to acknowledge the Wurundjeri, traditional owners of the land where this book was written and first published, and where the events take place. I would also like to pay respect to their elders, past and present, and extend that respect to other Aboriginal people reading this book. I thank Aunty Jacqui and Charley Woolmore from the Wurundjeri Tribe Land & Compensation Cultural Heritage Council for cultural advice.

Some people need someone to teach them how to listen, and for this I am grateful to Maggie Bolton. Some writers need someone to tell them to think of themselves as a writer, and for this I thank Lauren Berlant.

A writer is fortunate if they have a friend who is smarter than they are and who is prepared to read their work. If said friend is in possession of an unerring critical eye, an almost-always appropriate sense of humour, and has already published a book of their own, the writer is indeed very fortunate. I have such a friend: Anna Poletti. Whilst never reticent to tell me exactly what is wrong with what I've written, she is also able to tell me what's right with it.

What enabled me to get the writing done — and redone — was Anna's belief that this book was not only possible, but necessary and important. During one especially dark moment, when I had written only half a book and saw no way to write the other half, she asked me, 'If *you* don't write this book, who will?' It was then that I realised the simple fact that if I wanted this book to exist, I would have to *do* the writing. And I did it, but I owe Anna an immense debt of gratitude.

A writer needs a good editor, and I was fortunate in having two other acute minds generously apply themselves to the text in its final stages of becoming a book: my publisher, Henry Rosenbloom, and the late, great John Hirst. Whilst ensuring, through their thoughtful comments and insights, that I knew the emerging book was good, they let me know in no uncertain terms what needed changing for it to be publishable.

John Hirst was not only my editor and my agent by default; he was my champion. John believed in this book. He would read pages of the manuscript aloud to his friends and family, and to his students. He would report back enthusiastically how they laughed in the right places or were profoundly moved by one or another passage. It was this enthusiasm and his persistence that got me over the line. John's sudden death a few months before the book was due to be published was a shock and a huge loss. Like many others, I will miss his unwavering support, his wise counsel, and his unfailing bullshit detector. I am glad that he knew how grateful I was to him.

Last but certainly not least, I am indebted to Anna Thwaites at Scribe who came in at the eleventh hour and, with her sensitive edits, made the book so much better than it would have been. Scribe has a dream team in both hemispheres. I feel privileged to be published by them. Thanks to all of you.

I would also like to thank Ali Alizadeh, Robert Cane, Ceridwen Dovey, Anna Fienberg, Melinda Harvey, Nikki Morrison, Catherine Ringwood, Keith Stott, and Petra Watson-McNamara, who read early drafts of parts of the book and gave me encouragement and advice.

I especially wish to acknowledge the staff of the hospital, in particular the workers in the pastoral-care department who welcomed me, despite my unconventional approach to the work. To do justice to the importance of the friendships, support, and generosity of my colleagues and fellow interns in pastoral care would require a whole separate book. Maybe I'll write it one day. In the meantime, you know who you are, and I am grateful to you.

Most important of all, I want to thank the people who were in the hospital for treatment, their friends and partners, their sons and daughters, mothers, fathers, and other family members who shared their stories, their hopes and dreams, their regrets and their despair—including those who told me to go away. Without these people, this book would not exist.

Finally, to all the people who allowed me to talk about the book and the ideas in it along the way, I thank you for your friendship and your support, and wish you strength and wisdom in the difficult times ahead.

(The draft version of *I Am Here* began with a text by Mark

Linkous, comprising the lyrics of a Sparklehorse song called
'Sea of Teeth' that consoled me and inspired me during the
events I write about in the book—and still does. I was not
able to get permission in time to reproduce the lyrics, but you
can listen to the song here: bit.ly/sea_of_teeth)